The Branded Eye

The Branded Eye
Buñuel's *Un Chien andalou*

Jenaro Talens

Translated by Giulia Colaizzi

University of Minnesota Press
Minneapolis
London

The University of Minnesota Press gratefully acknowledges translation assistance provided by the Program for Cultural Cooperation between Spain's Ministry of Culture and United States Universities.

Originally appeared as *El ojo tachado*, Ediciones Cátedra S.A., 1986.

Published by the University of Minnesota Press
2037 University Avenue Southeast, Minneapolis, MN 55455-3092
Printed in the United States of America on acid-free paper

Library of Congress Cataloging-in-Publication Data

Talens, Jenaro, 1946–
  [Ojo tachado.   English]
  The branded eye : Buñuel's Un chien andalou / Jenaro
  Talens ; translated by Giulia Colaizzi.
    p. cm.
  Rev. ed. and translation of: El ojo tachado. 1986.
  Includes bibliographical references and index.
  ISBN 0-8166-2046-6 (alk. paper)
  ISBN 0-8166-2047-4 (pb : alk. paper)
  1. Chien andalou (Motion picture) 2. Buñuel, Luis,
1900–1983
  — Criticism and interpretation. I. Title.
  PN1997.C464243T3513   1993
  791.43'72—dc20   93-3662
                                                                  CIP

The University of Minnesota is an
equal-opportunity educator and employer.

La cinéma, disait André Bazin, substitue à notre re-
gard un monde qui s'accorde à nos désirs.

Jean-Luc Godard, *Le mépris*

Contents

Note to the English Edition

I finished writing this book in 1986. Since then, access to new bibliography and the analysis of other films by the director have led me, if not to a revision, to a nuancing of some of my statements and to some theoretical clarifications of the kind of reading that grounds them. This forced me to some changes: I rewrote the Introduction, and added several pages and numerous bibliographical references, which I hope have helped to clarify my position from a theoretical standpoint. All this, however, does not modify the scope and meaning of the Spanish version of the work, published by Ediciones Cátedra in 1986. The changes regard especially the use of certain concepts. I also have added some data and revised sentences that, read some time after the original writing of the text, might have been somewhat confusing. All translations of foreign-language source material are the work of the translator of this book, unless citation is given to a published English source.

I wish to thank Silvestra Mariniello for allowing me access to the manuscript of her book *Lev Kuleshov*. The lucidity and radicality of her analysis, especially with regard to a materialist understanding of filmic discourse, have been of great help in the development of some points that were only outlined in the previous version of my work.

Minneapolis, January 1989

Acknowledgments

A first, shorter version of the analysis of the first sequence of *Un Chien andalou* was delivered at the Universidad Internacional Menéndez y Pelayo in Santander, during the seminar on discourse analysis directed by José Luis López Aranguren and Jorge Lozano in August 1982.

The first chapter was partially published in *Eutopías*, vol. 2, no. 1, as part of the monographic issue on *Methodology of Image Analysis*.

In its present version the book is the result of a workshop held at the Center for the Humanities at the University of Minnesota in May 1984.

Tom Conley, who at the time was undertaking a similar project on *Land without Bread*, discussed my theses and provided me with a 16 mm copy of the film, taking up the ungrateful task of making the photographs of what was to become the first outline of the complete découpage of the film. Vicente Domingo later completed the task with a video copy and plenty of time and patience, in spite of the difficulties of working with video material (framing, darkening, low contrast, and so on), which made his efforts to obtain acceptable images twice as praiseworthy. He and Sergio Talens reviewed the film over and over again at the moviola with me and helped me double-check each of the photograms in appendix 2; they stoically put up with my finding out at each new revision that I needed more photograms or had to repeat some. My debt to them is enormous.

Gonzalo Abril, Juan-Miguel Company, René Jara, Thomas E. Lewis, Jorge Lozano, and Michael Nerlich also discussed with me parts of the text, although the final result is my total responsibility.

My thanks to all of them.

Valencia, January 1986

Introduction

In the opening scene of Ramón del Valle-Inclán's *Los cuernos de don Friolera*, Don Estrafalario, the prototype of the Valleinclanesque character, claims the right of an art capable of seeing the world from the other shore, with the same sarcasm and skepticism with which the dead look at the pedantic insignificance of the living.

With the exception of Valle-Inclán, rarely has this metaphor been used to articulate an artistic device with as much rigor as by Luis Buñuel, who makes an explicit reference to the world of the dead in the last lines of his autobiography, *My Last Sigh*:

> Frankly, despite my horror of the press, I'd love to rise from the grave every ten years or so and go buy a few newspapers. Ghostly pale, sliding silently along the walls, my papers under my arm, I'd return to the cemetery and read about all the disasters in the world before falling back to sleep, safe and secure in my tomb. (256)

For almost half a century, from *Un Chien andalou* to *That Obscure Object of Desire*, Buñuel's films have attempted, with admirable constancy and radicality, to question not only the cinematic apparatus itself — the mise-en-scène of a supposedly neutral and objective gaze — but also the incoherent logic that the imperialism of reason imposes on the real.

By means of an iconoclastic style and, in some way, against the grain of what can be broadly defined as mainstream cinema — within which the avant-garde would be but the other side of the institutionalized narrative mode — his work as filmmaker centered on a systematic attack of the optimism that founds the bourgeois vision of the world; his aim was to force the spectator to question the permanence of the established order and of the value system that supported it. This is the reason why his work focuses less on the supposed contents of each film than on the rhetoric of the discourse itself. In effect, if there is something that allows the establishment of a continuity between those films the director considered his personal films and the more commercial ones, it is an identical will to construct an equally critical gaze, even when using conventional raw materials.

This constancy has usually been defined in terms of faithfulness to his sur-realist beginnings, by taking for granted that his work belongs to a theoreti-cal and normative universe with which he actually was in touch only tangen-tially and ephemerally, and more for personal sympathy than for a real agreement with its principles.

Indeed, if a key date is to be located in Buñuel's biography, it is not the moment when he came into contact with the Parisian surrealists, but when he entered the Residencia de Estudiantes in Madrid in 1917. Many of the young Buñuel's attitudes (which we could define as dadaist, even though they have never been labeled as such), were common currency among some of the most progressive members of the new generation, under the evident influence of Ramón Gómez de la Serna and of Pepín Bello. Buñuel's staying in Paris would make many of these attitudes look "natural," but they had character-ized his behavior for a while before that. The fact that when he was a student in Madrid he disguised himself as a Prado museum guide and caused aston-ishment among the innocent visitors with his absurd comments about the paintings, or that in Paris he went to the premiere of his first film with his pockets full of rocks, prepared to defend himself from criticism, have been interpreted as surrealist gestures because of their similar provocative charac-ter. I believe, on the contrary, that these and other similar anecdotes should be considered as symptoms of a subversive, and not merely transgressive, viewpoint. It is indeed this subversiveness that distances his discursive prac-tice from the postulates of the Bretonian group, less concerned by the use-value than by the exchange value of such manifestations.

A reading of Buñuel's first film as a merely transgressive work may seem to be corroborated by the fact that the viscounts Charles and Marie-Laure de Noailles decided to finance also his first sound film, *The Age of Gold*. This was quite unusual, surprising both the Parisian aristocrats and intellectuals of the time, because, unlike the viscounts' collaboration with Manuel de Fal-la, it implied the acceptance and normalization of a certain idea of trans-gression — although not going beyond, however, what we could define as (to paraphrase García Berlanga in *Plácido*) "having a vanguardist sit at your table." The scandal that arose out of the film's premiere and the following incidents that brought the case to the French House of Representatives con-vinced the two sponsors, frightened by the general commotion, to withdraw all the existing copies of the film, including the original negatives. These would be recuperated for public viewing only in later years.

The making of Buñuel's next film was also characterized by similar limit-ing factors. He managed to shoot *Land without Bread* with money collected among his friends Ramón Acín, an anarchist and elementary school teacher in Huesca, poet Pierre Unik, cameraman Eli Lotar, and professor Sánchez Ventura. The film opened without sound track in 1933 at the Madrid Press Building and provoked a generalized indignation in the audience. Among the spectators was Gregorio Marañón, an intellectual who could be easily classified as one of the old "putrefied" from the student residence hall, capable of not giving *Lazarillo de Tormes* its due because he believed that its vision of Spain had contributed to the Black Legend. According to various accounts, the showing of the film caused an argument between Buñuel and Marañón, who could not tolerate the merciless representation of Spanish reality that the film presented.

Buñuel would not be able to savor again the taste of the financial and ideological independence of his first three films, at least not until the 1970s. Even then, it would be due more to the exchange value of the "auteur cinema" in the international market than to a real acceptance of his theoretical presuppositions. The films he made in this lapse of time are characterized by an apparent (and false) submission to the rules of classical narrative discourse and to the attendant structural model. Max Aub expressed this clearly in *Conversaciones con Buñuel*:

> Buñuel is not God; which means that he exists. Well, who knows. But I know gods exist: Picasso, for example; or Leonardo, Shakespeare, Cervantes. You feel that in whatever they touch. There may be doubts and especially imitations. This does not happen with Buñuel. He made a lot of movies that don't seem to be his—he was aware of that—in order to support himself. None of them, as he himself underlined, betrays his vision of the world, but it does not give it either. Like the work of every real creator, his work is not very large from this point of view, yet it is enough. The problem with Lope, with Federico, had he lived longer, is a different one: like Picasso, they were gods, but also squanderers. In their case a line, a detail was enough to reveal their genius. It is different with Buñuel: he ties himself to each one of his works with a determined spirit, "This is to eat" (and it is enough for it to be decent, in a bourgeois way) or "This is going to be part of something I have inside." The same thing has happened to all of us. Unless one prostitutes oneself, as Dalí did.

At the basis of Aub's comments, however, is an understanding of the thematic universe as the central axis of discourse. To some extent his words seem to imply that a point of view manifests itself in the (re)presented world, rather than in the gaze that grants that world status of (re)presentation. The perspective adopted in the present book questions this assumption. It is evident that every critical enterprise operates more easily in a setting where the possibility of choice is the widest; but if this critical project as such intends to affect the cultural debate at large or the social reality of which it is part, the so-called creative freedom has to be understood as submitted to the other discourses with which it conflicts and interacts. The conjunction character of every discursive practice is thus the necessary condition for the very existence of such practice. If this is what happens in the literary domain, for instance, it is much more evident in the case of cinema, whose industrial basis and market structure impose ineludible limitations. In this sense the difference between Buñuel's first three films (over which he had total control, as the director, screenplay writer, and producer) and the "commercial" ones of his Mexican phase is not particularly relevant to our purpose. In Aub's book, Buñuel himself affirms that he made *Susana*, *The Adventures of Robinson Crusoe*, and *The Criminal Life of Archibaldo de la Cruz* simply because he was asked to make them and because he needed to work, otherwise the idea to make those films never would have occurred to him. This does not mean, however, that each of these films does not represent, like the early ones, a similar ideological standpoint and an equally refined filmic project. What changes is the type of discourse with which each text establishes a dialogue and confrontation. In the case of his early trilogy, the interlocutors are the avant-garde and cinema itself as medium; in the later films it is melodrama or popular comedy as established and institutionalized genre. What remains constant is the critical dialogue established in each film between these discourses. What matters is never the narrated story — in the case of *Land without Bread*, the subject matter of the plot seems to be submitted to the genre defined, after Flaherty, as "documentary cinema"[1] — but the idea of approaching the cinematographic medium as a way to read the real either by means of a narrative argument or by the filming of "real" elements. The juxtaposition between fiction/nonfiction is irrelevant here, because the question is not so much *to show the world* but *to analyze how this world is looked at* (that is, *constructed*) by the cinematographic apparatus.

As in the respective cases of Fritz Lang in his American phase, Billy Wilder, Douglas Sirk, or Alfred Hitchcock, with whom Buñuel's work connects, from this point of view, in more than one way, even though it is much more materialist and radical, Buñuel's notion of the cinematographic apparatus simulates an enunciative transparency, a sort of formal neglect, which does not correspond at all to the utmost precision with which his films are in reality articulated. This is true for all his work, from his despised Mexican movies to his last films. The apparent linearity of the plot and the systematic renunciation of any gratuitous effect in the mise-en-scène characterizing his work as a whole have hindered the elaboration of a coherent and consequent critical approach. Thus the recurring references to the world of dreams that periodically mark and distort his stories operate a double closure when they are defined as a residue of his supposedly vanguardist phase. On the one hand, the corpus of his work is understood as merely "provocative" cinema; on the other, his early trilogy is recuperated as an instance of dysfunction, and the radical project that it implied is set apart from the rest of his work.

The question is that the role of film criticism, if any, whether within or at the margin of the academic institution, is less to *clarify* the spectator's position than to *classify*, *reduce*, and, eventually, *annul* the signifying capability of a film by inserting it within the register of the comprehensible. Critical endeavors do not simply accompany the unending flux of sense by describing its sources, they also attempt to channel it within the limits of what is considered to be the norm.

An explicit processual unity can nonetheless be identified in Buñuel's career as filmmaker, and this unity allows the study, from various perspectives, of his first three films and also others as different from each other as, for example, *The Young and the Damned*, *The Exterminating Angel*, *Cela s'appelle l'aurore*, and *Simon of the Desert*. This unity is based on Buñuel's peculiar notion of realism, which has allowed that, for nearly half a century, one of his films in particular has resisted all attempts to approach it analytically, even though its contradictory and irreducible simplicity offers a multiplicity of interpretive keys that exceed its value as individual work. In spite of its sixteen-and-a-half-minute length, *Un Chien andalou* still remains one of the most polemical and controversial movies in film history, apparently less "explicable" than *The Age of Gold* or *Land without Bread*.

The "real" is always inexplicable. "Reality" (or what we define as such) is not merely what *is*; it has been constructed beforehand as an explication. Each fragment has a logic and a function because it occupies a determined place so that the everyday chaos can function as a harmonious whole. Nothing is falser than realism in its traditional sense. From the beginning of his career, Buñuel took this principle as his point of departure and systematically denounced and denied realism's pretense to represent the truth in every single film he made, even in the most "documentary" of all, *Land without Bread*. The pessimist's logic belongs to the realm of conventions; the logic of the tragic terrorist that Buñuel was belongs to the realm of the absurd. The great lesson we learn from the filmmaker from Calanda is the necessity to assume this truth. His films are the splendid testimony of a tour de force: a type of realism that does not *reflect reality redundantly*, but *inscribes the real symbolically*. To approach *Un Chien andalou*, therefore, implies not only dealing with a specific text, but above all reflecting upon and reformulating what *reading a film* means.

The beginning of film theory in the 1920s, more than marking a point of departure in the elaboration of the instruments through which one could analyze an already-existing practice—cinema—meant the structuring of said practice as a controllable object, as readable from the perspective of the so-called arts that had been institutionalized by the bourgeois tradition. The invention of the term "seventh art" to describe cinema is not casual at all.[2]

Early cinema, in fact, has little to do with what its institutionalization as artistic discourse decided to fix in the second decade of the century. Today film historians speak of Porter, of Griffith's establishment of narrative rules, of Kuleshov's experiments, of the editing within the shot of expressionist cinema, or of Eisenstein's vertical editing. They speak, in short, of a series of technical procedures as bases for the periodization of cinema as language. Its development is thus historicized in such a way that one forgets that for the mass audience cinema addressed, what mattered was to go and watch a movie starring Douglas Fairbanks, Mary Pickford, or Lillian Gish, rather than a movie directed by David Griffith or Fred Niblo.[3] That is to say, one overlooks that the notion of "author" as support and sender of certain contents simply did not exist in early cinema. Film history as a discipline chooses as central axis of its own discourse the technosyntactical development of narrative cinema, which therefore became not one of cinema's dominant forms, but cinema *tout court*. In this way one elides, on the one hand, the whole problematic of the cinematographic spectacle as mass phenomenon and, on the other, all those proposals that did not submit themselves to the established models and rules of narrative logic. The differences between the various ways to understand filmic discourse can therefore be defined as different forms to approach narrative, an already-established and institutionalized genre in literature. It did not happen by chance that the first texts that attempted to address the new phenomenon—those by Hugo Munsterberg and Rudolf Arnheim—do not deal so much with the cinematographic medium as with its possible appropriation by philosophy or aesthetics.

In the case of those filmmakers inappropriately defined as "primitives," Lumière and Méliès especially, cinema did not mean a working-through of a notion of "reality" as referent to which the filmic object would refer one way or another, but a focus on the very material with which one worked.

The notion of "author" as sender of messages was diluted by and within the multiplicity of teamwork made necessary by the complexity of the technological production process. At the same time, the representational character of the word, or the line on the canvas in the case of painting, gave way to the physical presence of the filmic object. The text's relationship with the reader-spectator was therefore established on a different basis.

The subsequent development of the medium and its gradual utilization as "translator" of previous discourses[4] turned these pioneers into "primitives," because it was taken for granted at that point that the logical development of the new medium was that of narrating stories. The object film was thus defined as narrative and its revulsive potential as mass phenomenon foreclosed.[5] Noël Burch (1981, 1987) has provided an accurate and well-documented analysis of this process in the American cinema through the elaboration of what he has called the "institutional mode of representation" (IMR).

Silvestra Mariniello (1989) does something similar with Soviet cinema when she analyzes Lev Kuleshov's work. The director of *The Extraordinary Adventures of Mr. West in the Land of the Bolsheviks* has been inscribed in canonical film histories under the label of a technical experimenter, as the inventor of the so-called Kuleshov effect. With such a label, Mariniello points out, a double reduction has been accomplished: on Kuleshov himself and on the very notion of cinema that his work foregrounds. People have thus come to ignore that his work as filmmaker centered mainly on a relentless analysis of the dialectical relationship between the cinematic medium and the process of discursive production, rather than on the production of filmic objects. Moreover, a specific moment within the open process of investigation is turned into a constructive principle; by isolating it from the overall project, it is classified merely as an abstract technical device. The result of this twofold operation is the reintroduction of what Kuleshov always fought against: the distinction between form and content, a dichotomy that never worked as such in his work. For Kuleshov, as for Buñuel, the space of filmic discourse cannot be reduced to the production of a filmic object. It constitutes instead a mobile continuum, produced within the dialectical interaction between cinema and reality on the one hand, and between film and reading-appropriation on the part of the spectator on the other. What matters is not the finished and edited film, but the social process of meaning production within which the film's presence is inscribed, and the dialogue such process provokes. For this reason, for Kuleshov as for Buñuel, cinema as collective practice meant at the same time the end of art as it had been understood within bourgeois tradition—as analyzable only within the individualized and preestablished circuit author-reader—and the possibility of a new way to create a materialist mass spectacle. Mariniello points out how for Kuleshov the possibility to construct, for example, a human body as an effect of editing with pieces from different bodies without erasing the reality of the material was important not as a technosyntactical experiment, but because the spatio-temporal continuity established through editing allowed the articulation of a new relationship between cinema and reality, thanks to the establishment of a new form of perception. As we shall see later with the analysis of the opening sequence of *Un Chien andalou* and, even more explicitly, in all of his works following *Land without Bread*, Buñuel worked on the basis of similar presuppositions. From this perspective, Eisenstein's work, more than being a step ahead of Kuleshov's, meant the reintroduction of the bourgeois model of representation into filmic practice through the notions of "author" and "art," and the definitive support for the institutionalization of cinema as it is still conceived of today by critical discourse.

The institutional mode of representation thus took for granted the existence of a previous, punctually structured message in cinematic discourse, which assigned filmic material the mere function of a mode of articulation, the function of marking a style, or a form—no matter how elaborate. It produced the message as an effect and, by freezing the process as object, it located the spectator once more in the imaginary space of a passive receptor, a receptor on whom the mechanisms inherent to the film would act in a more or less indirect way; in short, a receptor that is manipulated from a different angle and with a different aim, yet still manipulated.

Mariniello (1992) quotes from Pasolini's 1966 essay "The Crisis of the Avant-Garde":

> Cinema does not evoke reality, as literary language does; it does not copy reality, as painting does; it does not mime reality, as drama does. Cinema reproduces reality, image and sound! By reproducing reality, what does cinema do? Cinema expresses reality with reality. If I want to represent Sanguineti, I do not resort to magical evocations (poetry), but I use Sanguineti himself. Or if Sanguineti is unwilling, I choose a long-nosed seminary student, or an umbrella salesman, in his Sunday best; in other words, I choose another Sanguineti. In any case, I do not go outside the circle of reality. I express reality—and therefore I detach myself from it—but I express it with reality itself.[6]

Buñuel's position does not differ much from Pasolini's, even though the concept of reality in Buñuel's filmic practice also includes the universe of the irrational and of dreams. In these terms it is possible to understand his difficulty with words, which was, in his opinion, what led to his devotion to cinema. The question is not so much his inability to *visualize* the world through verbal writing, but his resistance to inscribe a *presence* within a discourse that was traditionally based on *representation*; a question, in short, that concerns the material with which one works.

The contradiction between rationalism and irrationalism that characterizes much of the discursive production after romanticism finds in cinema a dialectical way to articulate itself. Méliès's first films, for example, play with magic (*The Famous Box Trick*) or science fiction (*A Trip to the Moon*). Yet, the rationality present in Méliès, because it has to be represented by means of a technological medium, shows how magic and science fiction are discursive effects, technical tricks—in short, rhetorical devices. No matter what Méliès's conscious intention was, we have an objective proof of the irrational as mise-en-scène; such is precisely what the institutionalization of cinema as art and narrative will later attempt to mystify by means of what has come to be known as the invisible editing. Cinema as craft could use elements from the so-called traditional arts, but in elaborating them by means of a different material and through the use of a technology irreducible to their logic, it could retrospectively reveal the false representational character of those elements. It could therefore show how referentiality is not a natural fact but a rhetorical construction. Perhaps this is why a theorization of cinema as technodiscursive medium can also cast light, in a more general way, on other discourses.

Buñuel stated in his conversations with Max Aub that for him the literary script was most important and that during the shooting he knew how to start but had no idea how each scene would develop.

Shooting is an accident, a necessary accident, so that others can see it. What matters to me is the setting, the script, the situations, the story, the dialogues. The word "camera" never appears in my scripts. I have no idea about the set, or of what exactly I am going to do. I don't have a schedule. I never know what I am going to shoot next . . . I know what the shot is going to be about, what is going to happen and what the characters are supposed to say, but I don't know what I am going to shoot first. Sometimes if in a sequence I feel that the actors enter and exit too much, I just frame something else and say something, or have the actor come in or go out, depending on what's needed. I do one take after another, with almost no editing needed. This is why the shots are never numbered and there are hardly any cuts in my films. I don't think it's really necessary to get any closer than a medium shot. Let me tell you: what matters to me is that the sequences as such say something, that they can be put to some use, that they get to the viewer without pretension. I never let anyone stay on the set at the end of the sequence. I usually spend a couple of hours thinking about the day's scene before the actual shooting. I know how to begin a sequence, but never how to end it.

Thus the term script cannot be understood as a literary argumental structure, but rather should be considered a basic system of relations. At the moment of shooting, plot, situations, and dialogues turn into mere raw materials that the physicality of the shooting can either assume or destroy, in accordance with the meaning that such physicality acquires through the cinematographic medium.

This system of relations allows the later elaboration of another system of relations—a physical one—because of the presence of certain *real* people and objects on the set. The juxtaposition of these two systems determines the effect of formal openness and disjointedness of most of Buñuel's films. We find in them an explicit refusal to objectify the mobile and changeable flux of discursive reality by foreclosing it. Such flux is produced by the dialectical relationship established among (a) the compositional formal material, (b) the plot's anecdotal subject matter, and (c) the physicality of the elements through which the former and the latter are articulated and shaped in the film. These elements are not subjected to each other hierarchically. Consequently, one cannot speak of formalism—the negative aspect weighing down the avant-garde's work—or of an excessive preoccupation with the text's content. Buñuel's corpus is therefore, in a strict sense, neither the work of an aesthete nor that of a narrator. Few filmmakers have been as little interested in narrating stories as he was, even though stories are his films' points of departure at times. His lack of interest in narration determines the fragmentation and apparent lack of logic that repeatedly break the argumentative control of his films, as Buñuel himself acknowledged when speaking of *Un Chien andalou*:

> What they say about the lack of coherence in *Un Chien andalou* is just nonsense. If this were the case, I would have cut the film as an ensemble of flashes, clustered the various gags, and spliced the sequences at random: there was no reason not to do so. But *Un Chien andalou* is simply a surrealist film whose sequences are put together according to a logical order whose expression is determined by the order of the unconscious. Notice that: unconscious, reason, logic, order. When the dying man falls in a garden, he caresses the naked shoulder of a statue (of a woman). That is to say, this is the normal consequence of the fall, it would have been absurd if

the latter sequence preceded the former. We use our dreams—and this is all but new—to express something, not to display nonsense. The only absurd thing in *Un Chien andalou* is the title. (Aub, 1985)

Every time one of the three elements listed above varies, the relationship between them also changes and, as a consequence, so does the discursive form of the result. Here we have the difference between *Un Chien andalou* and Buñuel's Mexican films, for example, not that the former is a "surrealist" film whereas the latter are conventional narrative ones. Even the necessity to work with very bad actors (which at one point Buñuel experienced rather frequently) is incorporated and used in the film as a mechanism for denaturalization and enunciative distancing from the argumental support. In other circumstances such distancing or rupture of the narrative effect is produced through editing. In *This Strange Passion* (1953) there is a sequence in which Arturo de Cordova looks at his beloved with an almost angelical expression while a Schubert sonata is played on the piano. The relationship between the images on the screen and the sound track established by the institutionalized narrative logic would accept as normal the parallel between the sentimental music of the sonata and the enthralled gaze of the male character. Buñuel destroys the linearity of the sequence at the level of both the sound and image tracks by introducing a noise of crashing plates and by cutting the shot to show Arturo de Cordova moving toward an open door that allows us to see the servant who dropped the plates. There is no explication of the event; the servant simply dropped them. But, at a discursive level, the interruption of the sequence determined by the servant's appearance breaks the magic produced as a *natural* fact by connecting Schubert's music with the adoring gaze of the male character. The fragmentation operated by Buñuel undoes such relationship, showing it as a rhetorical construction. Likewise the often-quoted blasphemous reference to da Vinci's *Last Supper* in *Viridiana* is a break in the narrative logic to which the sequence as a whole seems to be subjected. In this sequence thirteen beggars appear—exactly the right number to recreate the scene from Leonardo's painting. But there had been only nine beggars in the film, and nothing explains either before or after this sequence where the extra four necessary for the scene came from. Fragmentation as antinarrative procedure—proposed as such from the very beginning in *Un Chien andalou*—is most explicit in *The Phantom of Liberty*. The different stories that constitute the plot of this film are strung together by the protagonists' gratuitous running into each other in the final shot of each of the different episodes, none of which has a direct relationship with the others.

In *That Obscure Object of Desire*, the splitting of the female protagonist into two different actresses, Carole Bouquet and Angela Molina, undercuts all possible effects of verisimilitude. Even though each of the two actresses represents a different aspect of the same character, their different physical aspects underline their rhetorical function within the film. What would have worked "naturally" in a literary text is shown as a construction because of the impossibility, proper to filmic discourse, to represent it. We find something similar in one of the few explicitly cinematographic works by Jorge Luis Borges, *Les Autres*, directed by Hugo Santiago in 1972. The film is about a father who ends up assuming his son's personality while attempting to understand the reasons for his son's suicide. The use of the same actor to play both father and son unbalances the perfect and coherent logic of the literary screenplay, introducing those little cracks of nonsense, to which Borges refers in *Otras Inquisiciones*, that make one aware of the falseness of a flawless and apparently solid structure.

The lack of discursive analyses about *Un Chien andalou*, their replacement by either allegorical interpretations or vacuously laudatory evaluation, ultimately reducing the film to the avant-garde's artistic fetish, has implied the film's isolation as cult object and has furthermore determined the neutralization of the subversive power of a proposal that, although based on similar presuppositions, is much more explicit in this film than in the rest of Buñuel's filmography. All this is not gratuitous but rather symptomatic of a way to historicize cinema that does not take into account that its own object is a historical construction produced as a result of a process of institutionalization. Such an approach forecloses at the same time the possibility to revise, through the mechanisms of filmic discourse, the procedures at work in other practices, such as literature, painting, or theater, and does not question the interpretive status that underlies the act of reading in a way consonant with said process of institutionalization.

Filmic discourse, as it functions in *Un Chien andalou*, gathers, problematizes, and finally denies the canonical workings of traditional artistic discourses by conflicting with the epistemological system that supports them, and thus to read this film also presupposes to deal with the more general problem of *how to read*, that is, *how to produce sense* from a given text.

This is the ground this text intends to explore.

Chapter One

Discursive Strategies and Production of Sense

The Reader's Irruption

Roland Barthes's *The Pleasure of the Text* (1975) opens with a reference to that strange character that, when dealing with a text, is afraid neither of mixing contradictory discourses nor of dissolving in the vertigo of such contradiction. This character, which the institutional apparatus would condemn as an outcast in the name of the supreme law of critical analysis, is the reader, this "antihero" that "takes pleasure" at the moment of reading. In a different text, referring to some photograms from S. M. Eisenstein's *Ivan the Terrible*, Barthes (1970) alludes to the existence of a "third sense." He defines it as "obtuse sense," opposed to the "obvious sense." It originates from the very materiality of the text as a signifier without a specific meaning; it questions the norms and evaluations of criticism as metatextual discourse, thanks to its inherent incapacity to submit itself *to*, or be articulated *by*, them.

I shall not engage at this time in an analysis of such statements. Their meaning will become clear as soon as we start dealing with our own experience as readers/spectators. What I want to underscore here is the appearance, for the first time in theoretical discourse and radically proposed, of a new element—the reader—understood as a strategy to approach the textual apparatus.

The undeniable steps forward made by formalist and structuralist thought in stressing the necessity to focus on the object itself, on the one hand, and on its articulated character, on the other, brought about both a methodological opening and an epistemological closure in critical discourse. In the attempt to avoid both psychologistic superficiality and sociological reductionism, formalism and structuralism turned the critic or reader into a sort of discoverer of hidden treasures—meanings—that are supposed to be somewhere, implicit, waiting for someone to bring them to light through the possession and control of specific codes. The procedures' exhaustive power of explication would thus substitute the process of sense production.

1

The analysis of Baudelaire's *Les chats* by Lévi-Strauss and Jakobson is a paradigmatic example of this. In a way, both forms of analytical approximations can be incorporated into the definition of formalism given by Dana B. Polan (1985): a kind of empiricism in search of a theory to justify it. The divisions and structures that one seems to encounter in a text are nothing but the inevitable consequence of the act of theorizing about that very text. The *work* on a text is never inscribed objectively *in* it; neither can it be approached, consequently, as one of the text's attributes. The hypothesis of theoreticians such as Stephen Heath and Gillian Skirrow (1977), according to whom "there is a *generality* of ideology in the institution, 'before' the production of a particular ideological position" (57; emphasis in the original) does nothing but grant the text—as inscribed in a specific institution—a power that the text has only at the moment of the reading.

The direction that New Criticism moved into was not all too different. Almost following what T. S. Eliot had said explicitly when he stated that the critic's task was to find bad reasons for what we believe instinctively, even though the finding of such reasons is also an instinct, the perfect critic was considered the one who showed *intelligence itself swiftly operating the analysis of sensation to the point of principle and definition*. Theory could be understood as an orderly way to superimpose certain constructive principles onto the immediate perceptual data.

Like the positions of some contemporary American theoreticians who are dazzled by Derrida's thought but unable or unwilling to share in the radicality of his views,[1] Barthes's proposals tend to turn the resources of interpretative work against the rigidity of methodological or linguistic conventions by attempting to erase the borders between literature and theory. In this way, semiotics (or, more exactly, a certain way to understand semiotics) and deconstruction are constituted as juxtaposed approaches to discourse analysis, as irreducible to one another. Only the alternation or substitution of a *closure* with what could be defined as *arbitrariness of opening* could resolve a problem posited in these terms.

There is another way to conceive of semiotics. According to this different notion, the point is no longer "to merely apply a theory of signs, but to understand signification as a process that takes place in texts where subjects emerge and interact" (Lozano et al., 1982). Therefore, if "a text—any text—is always a failed act of writing" and if "we carry it through ultimately only because of the absence of what we really want to talk about" (Company, 1986), it may be pertinent to investigate in what way the critic's *desire* can inscribe itself in the object of the critic's work and produce sense through this work without turning the object into a mere "pre-text." It is important to see how this can be accomplished without trespassing certain limits of pertinence while at the same time accepting, on the one hand, the existence of an external object, historically produced and inscribed as such in a dialogical-discursive and also historical network and, on the other, the ineludible subjectivity of the gaze that confronts it.

The question is therefore how to combine the necessity for analytical rigor with the real—and arbitrary—position of the critic. Emilio Garroni (1974) provides a first working hypothesis when he talks about the aesthetic object as an inherently heterogeneous one. According to Garroni (1979), the presence in the aesthetic object of different codes that operate simultaneously denies the discursive specificity of such object, while allowing the critic to elaborate sense through a contextualization at an implicit level of what is presented in the text as explicit context. His thesis, however, outlines the question without answering it, because he leaves as unquestioned given not only the undeniable existence of objective codes, but also, fundamentally, their operative functionality, together with the whole problematic such concept implies.

If the production of sense is based on the acceptance—implicitation—of explicit codes, such process is, in itself, codifiable (that is, formalizable) and the difference between meaning and sense, even though signaled, is reduced to the question of the place (explicit and implicit, respectively) in which each is located. The vertigo of pleasure Barthes referred to, which is neither rationalizable nor reducible to any normative whatsoever, and is evident to any reader/spectator not compulsively convinced of the need for a scientific alibi, remains eluded.

It would perhaps be useful at this point to redefine the notion that grounds the polemic to which we have been referring, and around which both theoretical positions have been articulated, namely the notion of *text*.

Text vs. Textual Space

Since the first activities of the OPOIAZ and of the Moscow linguistic circle, literary theory in particular and theory of discourse in general have functioned with a triple semiotic model. The first two of these models are based as much on the work of Ferdinand de Saussure as on the mathematical model elaborated by Claude Elwood Shannon and Warren Weaver in 1949. In both models the text is conceived of as an autonomous system of signification, either in terms of *writing* (the former model) or in terms of *message* (the latter model). The third model derives from the writings of Charles Sanders Peirce, and does not define the sign as an entity or consider it within a system of relationships. Rather, this third model deals with the problem from a quite different point of view: the analysis and description of the necessary conditions for acts, facts, and objects to function *as* signs. The first two models are inserted into what we could define in terms of semiotics of communication; they study meanings and procedures used by the producers of signs not only to act on other meanings and producers of signs, but also to be acknowledged and accepted among them. The third model opens up a new space: the semiotics of signification, which studies all the uses and patterns of behavior that turn into signifiers for the fact that they occur in a socialized context.

Since the late 1960s semiotics has no longer been considered, at least by the majority of those who practice it, as the science of signs, but has functioned as a critical practice. Insofar as its critical objectives can be defined as (a) communication, (b) the structures of communication, and (c) the discourses implied in the communicative act, semiotics seems to be bent less toward the study of signifieds than to the very process of signification. Two different positions, irreducible to one another, are articulated in such process: the position of the speaker and that of the listener. Both positions are implicated in the process and their dialectical confrontation produces both the transformation of the (objective) meaning into (subjective) sense, and the symbolic or symptomatic inscription of both. With the term "symbolic inscription" I mean that which derives from an intentional act of discursive explicitation, and which is therefore analyzable by means of a rational structure that can be formalized; with the expression "symptomatic inscription" I mean the production of "a language effect in the speaker. The symptom is a metaphor, the ciphered message of a *jouissance* that the subject can no longer repress and in which the subject cannot recognize itself either" (García, 1983).

Every human science always implicates the person that practices it (and semiotics is no exception) because every single scientific endeavor necessarily places those that carry it out in a determined area of knowledge, forcing them to choose between cultural options that, in turn, affect their process of investigation. This is how dominant ideology determines not only the models of communication but also the instruments used to analyze their structure and function. There are no neutral sciences; the myth of scientific neutrality is an ideological illusion that emerged with Renaissance "scientific man." If not even the so-called exact sciences can ignore this principle, the myth of neutrality shows its mendacity most clearly in those disciplines defined as "human sciences," because their ideological determinations are more evident. The position of the critic/reader/spectator is not, therefore, one of extraneity to the object; on the contrary, this particular position constructs the object as such to a great extent. This compels us to acknowledge that two distinct notions have been subsumed simultaneously and ambiguously under the same notion of "text," each one referring back to a specific reality and position. The first refers back to the given object, and the second makes of the object the result of the critic/reader/spectator's work in his or her effort to appropriate the object in order to reconstruct the presence of the Other in the object's interstices. We shall define the former as *textual space*, and use the term *text* for the latter.

The notion of textual space, developed elsewhere in more detail (Company and Talens, 1984), takes different connotations depending on whether (a) it is organized structurally within a beginning and an end (TS); (b) it is a mere proposal, open to various possibilities of organization and fixation (TS1); (c) it presents no organization and fixation (TS2), even though it can be transformed into either of the previous two. In the first case we have, for example, the TS "film," "novel," "short story," and so on. In the second case, the TS1 "drama," "musical score," and so on. In the third case the TS2 "nature" (readable as landscape through its transformation into "painting"), "conversation" (readable as dialogue through its inclusion as part of a "drama"), "love relationship" (readable as performance of a ritual), and so on. *Textual space* as a concept can therefore account for any activity or situation in terms of textuality. From this perspective, *text* would be the transformation of one given textual space into a specific sense for a specific reader in a specific situation. It is clear, therefore, that there are as many texts as there are readings.

This distinction allows us to distinguish methodologically between two positions that are spatially and temporally different and to describe their differences as articulated ones, which permits us, in turn, to approach the notion of reading not as an act of decoding, but as an uninterrupted process of production/transformation. The problems deriving from the existence of evaluative hierarchies of interpretation do not send back therefore to the real, but to the discursive field of ideology. Paraphrasing Lewis Carroll's Humpty Dumpty, we could say that the question of meaning—the goal of

those practices based on the act of decoding—is not resolved in the establishment of the opposition possible/not possible, but depends on where and
how power is located. Sense, on the contrary, because of its own gratuitous
and chance character, escapes this logic. The risk of arbitrariness to which
each deconstructive endeavor is exposed can be avoided if we keep in mind
that the space where the reader's work is articulated is, if not fixed, at least
staked out. The limits to the production of the object text are imposed by
the textual space.

Writing as Reading in Progress

The act of reading is not so much to discover the meanings that the object
presents us with as manifestation of the supposed intention of a supposed author, but the amount of work required for the production of sense within the
framework in which such meanings are inscribed. In short, the question is
not to transcribe the monologue that the subject (author) carries through
these meanings, but to establish a dialogue with the object itself (understood
not as a closed universe, but as a moment in the processual becoming of the
discursive network in which it inserts itself) insofar as the object is what
speaks to us and speaks for us in answering our questions. The position of
the subject responsible for the answer can therefore be conceived of as an
empty space, a place constructed by the confrontation between the object
and the reader.

A theoretical layout as the one outlined here implies necessarily the questioning of many key notions of a theory of interpretation, because, from the
point of view of textual analysis, terms like author, recipient, or referent do
not send back to entities that exist independently outside discourse. They
are, rather, simply textual inscriptions of a discursive operation or strategy.
This is what allows one to see the interconnectedness between, for example,
literature, criticism, and translation: three fields of knowledge that belong
to one single space, that of the so-called verbal art, yet seem to be substantially different. The borders between them are erased, as they are three differen-
tiated stages of one common process.

Let us think, for example, of the way a poet operates when writing a
poem. Within a textual space of the third kind (TS2), formed by a con-
glomerate of various material (lived experiences, experiences of which one

has read or has come to know culturally or through everyday occupations, unconscious memory, that is, what we call imagination or inventiveness, and so on), the poet organizes a preliminary text, T. Split between functions as writer and as reader, the poet approaches T (which now becomes for the poet TS) and produces a certain sense. This sense is thus inscribed as meaning, through what we call the process of correction, in what for a new reader (or in a new reading by the same reader) would work in turn as TS, and so successively. In such process the reader, not the author, corrects, i.e., produces sense. Author and reader are different discursive operations located in different spaces, even though they disguise themselves under the same name. The difference between the author/reader's reading and that of any other reader —this is the role played by the critic—does not reside in a different structuring of the reading itself but in its pragmatic execution: in criticism, the sense of a text is not incorporated as meaning to the poem's textual space. In translation, the sense of a text produces a new textual space. The notions of author, recipient, and referent are defined in this case, more explicitly if possible, in terms of an operation, for they are constituted as discursive articulations and not as reflections of supposedly real entities within the process of textualization.

The Cinematic Textual Space as Model Textual Space

It should not surprise, therefore, that film, of all art forms, was to determine the widening of the problematic of the textual space. Who speaks in a film? Literature allows a comparatively easy metaphorization—the speaking subject *can be read* as the real subject lending its name for the inscription of the object as author—but it is difficult to do the same when confronted with a collective work, as in the case of the filmic object. Director, producer, scriptwriter, editor, actors, light technicians, and others compete for a privileged position that ultimately belongs to all of them without exception and to no one in particular, because it is the articulation of each of their discourses that ultimately constitutes the speaking subject. Such articulation manifests itself in an explicit textual manner: the editing. The fact that the product's final responsibility falls on one or another of the parts involved in the filmmaking process, depending on the power granted to each one within the structure of the film industry, does not change the terms of the question, nor does it grant any one of such entities the status of author. Our working hypothesis can therefore be as follows: more than any other traditional art practice, film allows (a) a definition of the author in terms of textual construction, therefore extraneous to manipulations of a psychologistic type, and (b) an understanding of editing (in the sense of mise-en-scène) as speaking subject. Thus, we can explain a pattern common to directors who worked within the constraints of the institutional mode of representation even though they did not endorse them at all (for example, Luis Buñuel, Billy Wilder, Fritz Lang, Douglas Sirk, or a woman director such as Dorothy Arzner, quite exemplary in this respect): explicitly ideological presuppositions at the level of the script are transgressed, if not totally denied, by the mise-en-scène. Whether what is subverted is the meaning of the film as a whole [as in *Fury* (Lang, 1936), *All That Heaven Allows* (Sirk, 1954), or *Dance, Girl, Dance* (Arzner, 1940)], the very existence of film as discursive typology (Buñuel's Mexican films or Lubitsch's films, for example), or the spectator's system of values (as in most of Wilder's work), the *operation* that constitutes the work of contextualization constructs at the same time a subject/author, a subject/spectator, and a referential system from which to read, as *function*, the symbolic inscriptions of the real.[2]

The rhetorical mechanisms at work in other institutionalized discourses, like literature for example, are not much different, but the representational character traditionally granted to such discourses by criticism has not always permitted the acceptance of such principles in an approach to literary texts. From this perspective film analysis lets scholars return to literary texts with new instruments for reading that have made it possible to see those mechanisms in a new light. Juan-Miguel Company has shown this both in his book on Zola and realism (1986) and in his study of the relationship between realist writing and Hollywood cinema (1987).

Buñuel's *Un Chien andalou* situates itself explicitly in this perspective from the very beginning of the director's career as filmmaker. Before we turn to a detailed analysis of the film, we need to discuss two notions that are presented quite radically in the Aragonese director's first film: mise-en-scène as negation of the film's explicit meaning, and textual space as context. Yet, because *Un Chien andalou* may seem to constitute a separate case because of its supposedly "vanguardist" character, we will address these two concepts by briefly analyzing three films that are all considered exemplary of classical narrative although differing quite a bit from each other.

Mise-en-scène as Negation of the Film's Explicit Meaning

In our study of the first of these notions, let us consider two films, a comedy that belongs to the period of the Hollywood classics and a monumental melodrama: *To Be or Not to Be* and *Gone with the Wind*, respectively.

In *To Be or Not to Be* (Ernst Lubitsch, 1942) the openly erotic character of the relationship between the young aviator (Robert Stack) and the famous Polish actress Maria Tura (Carole Lombard) is relegated to an amiable background at the level of the script, in spite of the sexual ambiguity of the verbal exchange between the two characters during their first meeting in Maria's dressing room. The fierce satire of nazism articulating most of the argumental vicissitudes overshadows all other possible reading of the opposition life as desire (Carole Lombard/Robert Stack) vs. life as representation (Jack Benny), an opposition that pushes the film beyond the entertainment of the historical-metaphorical anecdote.

At the end of the sequence of the Shakespearean monologue, the shot of Hamlet/Joseph Tura (Jack Benny) looking with a puzzled expression at a young spectator leaving the theater (photogram 1) is linked by means of a fade to the beginning of the sequence in the dressing room (photogram 2). Thus the woman's (supposed) suitor enters the frame as if emerging from the phantasmic dissolution of the husband figure, whose place he will eventually take.

Without questioning the spatiotemporal relationship established by the fade, typical of the classical syntax in the Hollywood narrative model,[3] the

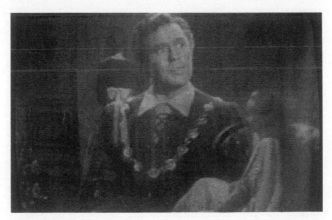

Photogram 1

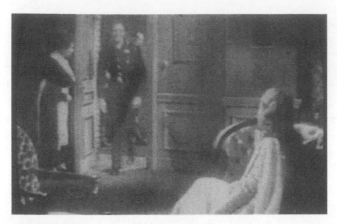

Photogram 2

film simultaneously inscribes a change in space and time and a symbolic index of what, from that moment on, will explain the characters' behavior. The whole beginning of the new sequence is shot from the space on the left of the axis that crosses the door vertically, leaving the woman (Ophelia / Maria Tura / Carole Lombard) to the right and the mirror and vanity in the offscreen space at the spectator's left (photogram 3). The staging of the sequence respects rigorously the 180-degree rule until the moment in which the young aviator states, with the swankiness of a naive lady-killer, that he is capable of dropping three tons of dynamite in two minutes from his bomber. The aviator's naive affirmation of power acquires at once a sexual undertone in the actress's ears. At that moment, and coinciding with Maria's

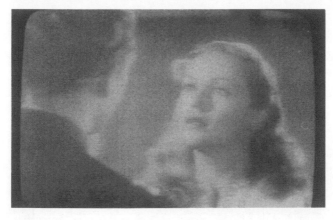

Photogram 3

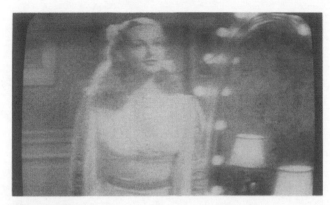

Photogram 4

sudden interest in her admirer, the camera breaks the 180-degree rule and frames Maria in a space that is physically the same, but where the (symbolic) positions of the two characters have changed. Maria, standing sideways before a mirror that reflects nothing (at least from the spectator's point of view) except for its utmost emptiness (photogram 4), is no longer the seductive *image* that received the aviator with customary indifference at the beginning of the sequence; she becomes instead the *symptom* of a real erotic desire. It is not by chance that when Maria asks her assistant what she thinks of the scene she has just witnessed, the woman comments that "what a husband doesn't know won't hurt his wife."

The new framing will be kept until the young aviator leaves the dressing room (photogram 5). The original framing returns with the following shot, when a cut shows the entrance of a depressed Joseph Tura, shaken by what

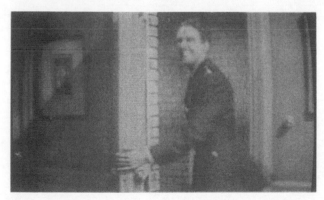

Photogram 5

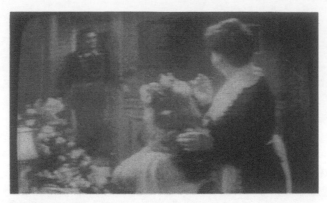

Photogram 6

he considers to be a sign of his decadence as an actor (photogram 6). Nothing has happened but the creation (meanwhile) of a *different space for a different relationship* explicitly situated, through the mise-en-scène, out of the husband's field of vision.

Something similar — although more radical in the wider opening-up of sense it produces — happens in the renowned *Gone with the Wind* (Victor Fleming, 1939). This classic melodrama is apparently a saga of the American Civil War years, but a different meaning emerges from the patent explicitness of the textual space through the staging of the events, which turns the film into what patriarchal discourse would define as the *history of a hysteria*.

The first thing to appear on the screen after the opening credits is a black man running after a fleeing turkey (photogram 7). A cut shows the stairs

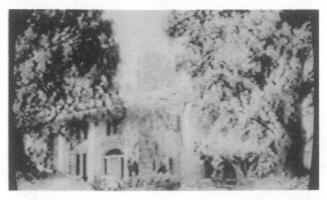

Photogram 7

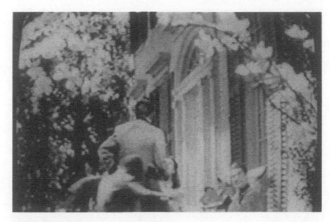

Photogram 8

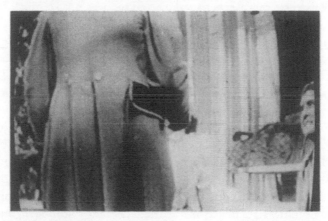

Photogram 9

where Scarlett O'Hara (Vivien Leigh) is being adored by the Tarleton twins, admirers of her beauty (and of her attendant unavailability). At this point the bird and its pursuer cross the screen from left to right (photogram 8), establishing a syntagmatic relationship with the scene developing in the background. Once the man and the bird disappear, the camera begins a slow tracking shot forward and the twins (one of whom gives his back to the camera) move aside, literally opening up the space between them as stage curtains (photogram 9). Next comes a close-up of Scarlett (photogram 10), who begins at this point to play the part of the seductress ("War, war, war!") with the serenity of one who is aware of being on stage and knows all the actor's

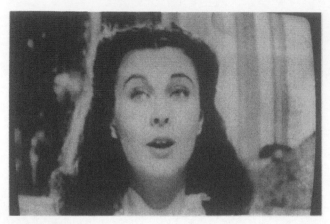

Photogram 10

tricks: the hysteric represents to seduce and seduces not so much to possess as much as to avoid being possessed.

The characters' subsequent development seems to follow such apparently insignificant beginning. The attraction Scarlett feels for Rhett Butler (Clark Gable), the only male character that does not immediately fall into the game's trap, is noticeable from the film's very beginning, even though this attraction will remain unacknowledged until the end of the second part. Rhett's presence seems to counter the dullness of Ashley Wilkes (Leslie Howard), first the fiancé and then the husband of Melanie Hamilton (Olivia De Havilland), a sort of mirror that returns Scarlett her own bodiless unavailability.

From the point of view of the film's traditional narrative support—the narrative meaning structuring it—Scarlett O'Hara's stubborn rejection of Rhett Butler can be easily explained by the impossibility of having him occupy a place that is taken up by another love (another image). In this case as well, however, the mise-en-scène establishes through editing a direct connection between elements that are equivalent positionally, turning such elements into bearers of a different implicit meaning.

In one of the film's early scenes Scarlett's father (Thomas Mitchell) talks to his daughter about the importance of land, of which Tara is a symbol, while they walk on the plantation grounds of Seven Oaks (photogram 11). Interestingly enough, the unreal quality of William Cameron Menzies's marvelous setting of the scene, with the pastel red of the background, appears

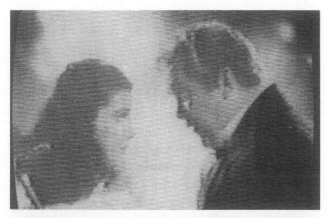

Photogram 11

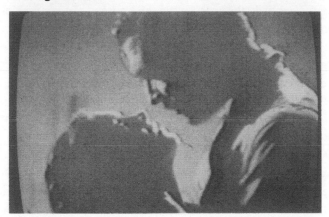

Photogram 12

again in the bridge sequence after the escape from Atlanta. In this scene Rhett Butler occupies the father's position (photogram 12).

The whole film is indeed traversed by Rhett's symptomatization of Scarlett's oedipal relationship to her father. Rhett seems to have the power to solve problems, a sort of superior strength one can rely upon; he is the exteriorized image of the understanding father, to whom Scarlett feels attracted (as image) and whom she rejects (as function) at the same time. The subtlety of the process is neither gratuitous nor casual. In the second part of the film, during the honeymoon along the Mississippi River, Scarlett wakes up in fright and recounts her nightmare to Rhett:

SCARLETT: Oh, Rhett, I was so cold and hungry . . . and so tired! I couldn't
find it! I ran through the mist but I couldn't find it!

RHETT: Find what, honey?

SCARLETT: I don't know. I always dream the same dream and I never know! It
seems to be hidden in the mist.

RHETT: Darling!

SCARLETT: Rhett, do you think I'll ever dream that I have found it—and that
I'm safe?

RHETT: Dreams don't work that way. But when you get used to being safe
and warm, you'll stop dreaming that dream. . . . And, Scarlett,
I'm going to see that you are safe. (Emphasis added.)

Having found out after Melanie's death that her ethereal lover never
really loved her, Scarlett turns to her husband—and discovers that he has
disappeared. Terrified, she goes out of the house—a heavy mist all around
her—and runs desperately up the hill, unaware of what she will find at the
end: Rhett's desertion. Exactly at the moment when the door closes behind
him and as Scarlett, who has thrown herself on the stairs, is confronted for
the first time with her real solitude (there are no spectators now, and thus
the representation that began in the sequence with the twins is over), we
hear her father's voice in the sound track repeating the same sentences he
uttered in the sequence at Seven Oaks. The (real) absence of the symbolic
father has been substituted by the (phantasmic) presence of the absent father. Again, the relationship established through editing between two of the
film's discursive fragments—although here the relationship is established between one element of the sound track and one from the image track—allows
the production of a sense that is not inscribed as meaning at the level of the
plot.

Textual Space as Context: The Referential Function

Having addressed the notions of author and reader/spectator as textual
products, we shall now deal briefly with the third element: the question of
the referent. What does a film speak about? In terms of textual analysis it
may be more productive operationally to substitute this question with another: from where does a film speak? A work such as *Raiders of the Lost Ark*
(Steven Spielberg, 1979) can be useful in dealing with this problem. Despite

or perhaps because of its extraordinary box-office success, the film has been too quickly condemned to the inferno of the kitsch, due also to the evident importance given by Spielberg to the cinephilic citation. I am not going to linger on a detailed analysis of what, in spite of everything, this film—rather peculiar in the director's trajectory—represents, in my opinion; neither shall I elaborate the reasons why I believe it at least deserves to be studied as exemplary of a position that is (readable as) critical of the cinephilia that grounds it.[4] I believe its very explicit appearance of pastiche makes *Raiders of the Lost Ark* interesting to talk about, because it makes a clearer reference than *Un Chien andalou* (an undoubtedly more complex work) to the universe of discourse as the place from where to read a film.

To begin with, a plot narrating Hitler's search for the Ark of the Covenant to strengthen the German army is undoubtedly a historical blunder. Such unreal and unrealistic anecdote—yet all but gratuitous within the film's logic—should be related to a whole series of other textual inscriptions meant to underscore the film's talelike quality.

The film opens with the logo of Paramount Pictures (photogram 13). From the logo's mountain another mountain emerges by means of a fade, a real one this time—within the fiction—on whose backdrop the characters move as the credits disappear from the screen (photograms 14 and 15). From the very first moment the film presents us with the explicit materialization of the fact that what we shall see originates, in a literal way, from a specific narrative tradition, the one established by Paramount in the course of its history.[5] Such declaration of principles would be nothing but a superficial wink,

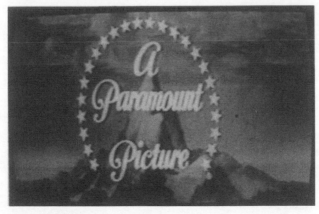

Photogram 13

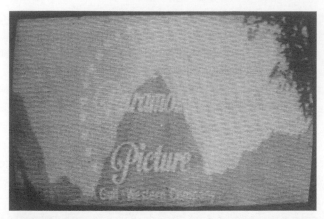

Photogram 14

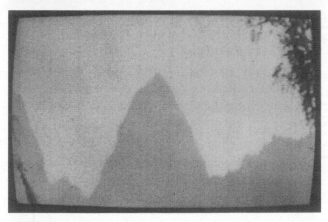

Photogram 15

were it not for the contextualization of the first two sequences-prologue it provides; they in turn contextualize the film as a whole. This may indeed be their only function, as the story of the "lost Ark" starts only with the third sequence.

Unlike classical films, which *Raiders of the Lost Ark* seems to imitate, there are no heroes here as such from the very beginning, destined to carry out their tasks, but instead there are stand-ins that only acquire body and consistency as a result of the tasks they carry out. During Indiana Jones's (Harrison Ford) escape through the forest we see his figure only in backlighting, in the shade, or from behind. When he snatches away with his whip the gun from the hand of one of the guides who is about to shoot him from behind, the camera zooms forward, finally revealing and showing us for the first time his face, moving toward the light.

This cold, calculating, and bold hero is characterized by his external attributes: a hat, a whip, a gun. The second sequence shows him in his role as a shy archaeology professor who hides his fear of the tricks of love behind glasses and a formal attire, even though his attractive figure affects equally both males and females. His students look at him with the air of a foreboding swooning; one has even written "I LOVE YOU" on her eyelid, and on his way out of class a male student leaves, almost in passing, the apple of temptation on top of the professor's desk.

The two fundamental features for the definition and believability of an adventurer as a "humanized" typology have already been given. They need only be articulated. At the end of the second sequence, once he has been officially put in charge of the search for the "lost Ark," Indiana Jones picks up his gun and whip—in two close-up inserts—and boards the plane to begin his adventure, impeccably dressed with a hat and a necktie. If the first two sequences made believable a character that from that moment on would act in accordance with the model they outlined, the verisimilitude of the adventure as such will be supported by the three shots we have just pointed out. Because we are watching a movie, and because everything is possible in film, it will not surprise us that the main character crosses the Pacific Ocean on the deck of a submarine and arrives at his destination, although a bit wet, in a perfectly healthy condition.

Reading as Construction of the Filmic Object:
Poetic Discourse vs. Narrative Discourse

From this brief analysis of examples from other films, we shall now move on to a thorough discussion of one more concept, indispensable, in my opinion, to an approach to Buñuel's film: the notion of *reading as construction*.

As we have just seen, a film's subject matter is not what decides the direction of the sense that the text proposes to the reader. We are therefore authorized to infer the necessity to differentiate two levels that superimpose each other but are to be kept distinct: (a) that which refers back to the film's subject matter, and (b) that which corresponds to the system of operations that articulate the film's subject matter as structure.

In the former case, on the basis of a predicative act, the film's subject matter seems to point to an extradiscursive real as its referent; in the latter, each element refers back operationally to other elements within the immanence of the closed system that constitutes the textual space. Both levels offer signifying elements to the spectator: the first level in an immediate and cumulative way; the second one through composition and from the end, by assuming all partials signifiers and signifieds (if there are any) and connoting them retrospectively, without ever being confused with them. Denotations and connotations thus accumulate. Connotations amplify and recuperate denotations, incorporating them into their own system. What matters is the signifying opening produced in the specific actualization of discourse, because discourse as such is less representative of the world than of itself; it is therefore neither a projection nor a description of the real, and not even a commentary on it (certainly not its repetition either). "To read" a textual space, then, means to establish its meaningful borders, elaborating—differentiating—the three levels of the signifying process that constitute its explicit context.

We shall call the first level signification A; it is produced by the basic elements used as raw material. In the case of the film we are discussing, this corresponds to a number of images dialogically connected to a wide spectrum of cultural, iconographic, and literary referents to which *Un Chien andalou* hints explicitly, as Aranda (1969), Morris (1972), Conrad (1974), and Drummond (1977) have indicated. Among these images mention should be made, for example, of Dalí's work (to which Drummond refers in connection with the segment of the two pianos), Buster Keaton's films, and also a large number of literary figures, thought of as untouchable until then, but considered by the scriptwriters as exemplary figures of the "putrefied."[6]

The second level, signification B, is produced both by the concrete articulation of these elements and by their inscription into a specific discursive typology. Both cases involve a process of coding/decoding, that is, the production of messages that are subjected to codes.

The third level, signification C, corresponds to a noncodified symbolic signification that, in implicating us as real spectators, allows us to appropriate, that is, experience it, as something we interiorize and identify with. This third level of signification allows the production of sense that we previously mentioned. If the conditions for discursive production base their verisimilitude or intelligibility on what we have defined as significations A or B, the disappearance or spectatorial lack of control of the corresponding codes necessarily implies for the reader the impossibility to determine a specific sense. If, on the contrary, this happens in the case of signification C, the production of sense will not only be possible, it will represent the only viable way to *construct* some kind of intelligibility for the object that embodies such intelligibility.

In the case of *Un Chien andalou*, the two processes we have defined as significations A and B are subjected to the third typology because of the way such typology transforms an apparently narrative apparatus into a poetic one.

What I mean with these two categories are distinct articulations of discourse, not differential categories at the level of content. An initial hypothesis could be enunciated in the following terms: the narrative apparatus, whose most concrete manifestation is the traditional narrative ("Once upon a time"), is based on the temporal relationship of events someone narrates and articulates; the poetic apparatus is based on the very process of articulation, which is in itself the only narrated event, or at least the main one. What will differentiate the two typologies is something internal to the object in which discourse is actualized and carried out—that is, the different mechanism that constitutes it—but also and fundamentally the different relationship established between such mechanism and the spectatorial subject that confronts it.

As far as the first distinction is concerned, the articulation of the events in narrative discourse takes place within a logic that makes them believable. Such believability is based on the displacement of temporality toward causality. It is therefore a twofold determined structure. Barthes (1966) pointed this out when he analyzed the effect of sequentiality in narrative: what comes after something else (in succession) is confused with the logic of causality (as a consequence). For this reason the conditions for narrative closure in the institutional mode of representation are already inscribed in the narrative's very beginning (Kuntzel, 1972).[7] In poetic discourse, this articulation is not subjected to events; it is not fortuitous in the sense that it does not constitute a self-enclosed universe, but a succession of fragments. In the same way the characters embody the logic of causality of narrative discourse: they are constructed as psychologically motivated and provided with traits befitting the narrated story line. This type of construction is missing from the discourse defined here as poetic. Finally, in narrative discourse the spatiotemporal dimensions (space on the screen and duration) represent the space and time of the events in the narrative chain and are therefore subordinated to the space and time of the narrated story. Narrative space is thus a scenographic space within which actions are framed as events. Narrative time is constituted as elliptic time either to allow the progression of the story or to explain the motivations for the characters' actions. Space and time are thus subordinated to the logic of causality. Such subordination is not pertinent to poetic discourse.

About the second distinction we have made, it should be noted that, in narrative, sense is produced through the elaboration of the meaning of present elements; in poetic discourse this is accomplished through the elaboration of the nonmeaning of absent elements, that is, by means of the fissures between links. The spectatorial function in narrative is a merely intellectual and passive presence; in poetic discourse, it is also a sensitive and necessarily active presence. In narrative the reader/spectator has to discover and recognize; in poetic discourse the reader/spectator has to construct, that is, (re)cognize. This is what distinguishes Joyce's *Ulysses* from Beckett's *Comment c'est*, Velázquez's *The Surrender of Breda* (*Las lanzas*) from Casimir Malevich's *White on White*, Howard Hawks's *The Big Sleep* from Buñuel's *Un Chien andalou*, with no value judgment implied. Precisely because of the greater amount of freedom characterizing the spectatorial function of poetic discourse, because of the ability required to use the codes without being submitted to them, because of the possibility it provides to produce messages without a preestablished code, poetic discourse has to do with subversion.

Subversion, as Mikel Dufrenne (1979) has shown, designates an action and its effect by stressing the effectiveness of the enterprise, not its nature or structure. It is, for this reason, an axiologically neutral term. It is positive or negative not in itself, but only depending on who utters it.

The notion of subversion, Dufrenne continues, is connected to that of system, understood not as a concept but as a word that denotes nothing specifically, but offers a vast range of connotations for concrete people by naming a lived experience or one that is possible in real life. Such experience tends to define as "system" all that presents an intelligibility and hostility similar to its own. It turns the term into something that hints to an undifferentiated totality that, when interiorized by an individual person, depersonalizes and erases that person rather than constituting him or her as a subject.

Such understanding of subversion leads us to a distinction between subversion and two concepts with which it has usually been associated: transgression and perversion. Contrary to subversion, transgressive and perverse practices presuppose the acceptance of the system they want to or say they transgress or pervert. Indeed, their relationship with the system constitutes their raison d'être, their survival depends on the survival of the system. Transgression is played as a dysfunction of the system and from within the very system that grants its stability, even though stability does not seem to be its objective. This is why transgression often takes the shape of marginality and becomes, like marginality, a form of order. Let us consider as example *M* (Fritz Lang, 1930). In this film the presence of the little girls' murderer jeopardizes life in the underworld because it prompts the police to investigate. This makes the slum dwellers function as a parallel police. Both police and the denizens of the underworld intend to maintain the established status quo, on whose weakness the latter thrive. Law and transgression thus go hand in hand within the same ideological territory.

Perversion also moves within the system, among the interstices of the logic that it attempts to exploit to its own advantage. In this case we may find examples in *Monsieur Verdoux* (Charles Chaplin, 1947) or *The Fall of the American Empire* (Dennis Arcand, 1987). Both the old Bluebeard protagonist of Chaplin's film and the bon vivants professors of Arcand's film play their parts on the preestablished ground of a double morality. They are at the same time honest citizens and consequent debauched. Their perverse practices belong to the order of morality, whose underpinnings they never really question.

Subversive practice pits itself against this very concrete "system." It does so not by attempting to trick its laws, as transgression does, or by seeking to reflect a mirror image of its morality, as perversion pretends to do. Subversion seeks to destruct those laws and to destruct with them the very system that engenders them and by which it is engendered.

In this endeavor, subversive practice is connected to revolutionary practice, although it cannot be identified with it. Subversion is punctual and not tactical; it eludes the systemic structure as all systemic discourse is at the same time an instrument *of* and *for* power. In relation to issues that are not of a strictly structural nature, however, subversive practice does not operate from a general theory of reality or of the system that constitutes it, but from the experience of human beings in that reality and those systems. Thus, its motor is not abstract thought, but desire; a desire understood not as *lack of being* but as *provocation to action*.

This is what I mean when I refer to the relationship between subversion and what I have defined as poetic discourse, between subversive practice and the processes of production and reading of poetic discourse. Poetic discourse is not only produced in a fragmentary manner, it also offers itself to reading by referring back to the fragmented body of the real, not by returning the false image of totality of which the structured order of narrative discourse consists. This situates the spectator in a place that is necessarily different from the one occupied by the spectator of Hollywood classical film because it individualizes the viewer and does not make of him or her a mere "individual representative" of the generic and systemic spectator that Hollywood classical film presupposes. If a general theory of narrative cinema is possible (and it has been done), a general theory of poetic discourse is less likely to be elaborated; the most it could accomplish would be to describe the operations taking place in specific objects, without ever being able to constitute itself as an analytical "model."

This should not prevent us, however, from attempting to describe a specific corpus of procedures that, without ever constituting a normative rhetorical system, allows the establishment of a set of parameters from which to approach Buñuel's filmography, which *Un Chien andalou* prefigures in such manifest way.

By saying this I do not pretend to invoke a Buñuelean "style," as a codifiable trademark, in the same way as one speaks of the "Lubitsch touch." Instead, I wish to point to the existence of a point of view rigorous as much as coherent, developed in the course of nearly half a century. The apparent formal "neglect" of such point of view is the implementation of a function that is metadiscursive and ideological at the same time, present in films so different from each other as *The Exterminating Angel* and *Viridiana*, or also in the so-called minor films, as *Subida al cielo* or *Susana*, submitted to the genre's or the industry's limitations.

It seems that the films where such mechanism is the most explicit allowed a false rhetorical codification of Buñuel's work and its recuperation, that is, the neutralization of their subversiveness and radicality on the part of dominant cinema. *The Age of Gold* took Buñuel to Hollywood; *The Discreet Charm of the Bourgeoisie* brought an Academy Award to a director whose work is totally irreducible to the industry's requirements and presuppositions.

This is the reason why his first short film is twice as important. First because, from the perspective we have already outlined, *Un Chien andalou* is the perfect example of the subversiveness of poetic discourse, even more than the already-systematized *The Age of Gold*, which it surpasses in terms of boldness and radicality. In *The Age of Gold*, Buñuel does not pillory, as Juan-Miguel Company (1983) pointed out, "any system of representation. It is a film made of narrative anecdotes in which some *symbolic enunciates* have been structured, the majority of which are particularly obvious, including the rudimentary class struggle apparatus by which the filmic discourse is supposed to be articulated." Second, because the utmost simplicity of *Un Chien andalou* places it very far from both the allegorical reductionism that has marked the failure of some of Buñuel's supposed disciples (Carlos Saura, for example) and the sometimes easy metaphoricity of some of his great admirers, like Alfred Hitchcock.

A discussion of why and to what point film industry, in spite of everything, has not been able to "recuperate" this type of practice would take us too far from the issues that are at stake in the present book. However, if it is undeniable that Buñuel's later films simulate a submission to classical narrative, it is also true that this submission allowed him to escape the "vanguardist" cliché that has afflicted, so to speak, many of the directors that today claim his *opera prima* as their reference point. Such submission also allowed him to offer a gamut of procedures easily detectable as textual inscription in directors as different from each other as Alfred Hitchcock, Roman Polanski, Pier Paolo Pasolini, or Samuel Beckett, to name only a few. As an example, let us refer to the last shot of *North by Northwest* (Hitchcock, 1958), where we can detect a clear relationship, perhaps anecdotically fortuitous, with the final shots of *This Strange Passion* (Buñuel, 1953).

In Hitchcock's film, Cary Grant stretches out his hand to prevent Eva Marie Saint from falling down one of the giant faces of Mount Rushmore. A cut shows a woman being pulled up by a man's hand, but now we are in a sleeping-car compartment. The following shot shows, in an obvious sexual metaphor, the train entering at full speed a tunnel in the background.

In Buñuel's film, the two main characters visit the woman's ex-husband, who was once obsessed with his wife's supposed unfaithfulness and now lives in his definitive madness in a Latin American monastery. A child is with the couple. When one of the monks asks the couple who the child's father is, the question remains unanswered. After they leave, we see the ex-husband weaving his way toward a dark doorway at the end of a path in the background.

Compared to the obviousness of the procedure and its functioning as an ornamental paraph in Hitchcock's film, Buñuel's mise-en-scène ends the film without closuring its sense; instead, it poses new questions that force the spectator to think over the story she or he has just seen. Although the series of events is diegetically explained in both cases, in the film by the Aragonese director the final shot is a return to the beginning rather than the film's closing moment; it multiplies the text's signifying possibilities by inscribing retrospectively in the film the equivocal ambiguity of its own interpretative codes.

Another example comes from the reminiscence—explicitly acknowledged this time—of the sequence of the slit eye of *Un Chien andalou* in the last sequence of Roman Polanski's *Chinatown* (1972). A bullet fired by the charac-

ter played by the film's director—as in Buñuel's film—shoots Faye Duna-
way's eye out of its socket. The relationship between the two films is very
superficial, however, because, as we shall see in chapter 2, the signifying value of the slitting of the eye in Buñuel's film has a much wider reach than in
Polanski's otherwise excellent thriller.

The intimate relationship existing between the thematic and argumental
issues of *Teorema* (Pier Paolo Pasolini, 1967) and *Susana* (Buñuel, 1950)
should be underscored. In Pasolini's film, the irruption of the problem-
raising character (Terence Stamp) is resolved with the father's undressing at
the train station, a sort of final, almost mystical self-purification; in Buñuel's
film, on the contrary, nothing is resolved. Susana goes back to prison, and
in the landowners' family everything continues as usual, stable in the same
decent putrefaction. The revolutionary reach of moral transgression, Buñuel
seems to imply, has its limitations.

We can trace Buñuel's influence on Samuel Beckett in *Happy Days*, where
Winnie is buried in the sand like the two characters in the final shot of *Un
Chien andalou*, which Beckett must have seen when he was a lecturer at Paris
École Normale. Unlike the previous three examples, however, this is not a
superficial quote, for Beckett picks up Buñuel's discourse and radicalizes it.
What in Buñuel's work constituted an arrival point becomes with Beckett a
point of departure.

These four brief examples point to the deep imprint left in film history by
a point of view whose fundamental features had already been outlined, in all
their radicality, at the very beginning of Buñuel's trajectory, in a short film
of sixteen and a half minutes. The film was made with a very small budget
and without the support of sophisticated technology, but with the intelligence and rigor of a person who knows very well what film consists of, not
only as spectacle but also and especially as writing.

Chapter Two
Reading of *Un Chien andalou*

An Irreducible Model

Un Chien andalou, made by Luis Buñuel in 1929 from a script the director wrote in collaboration with Salvador Dalí, is perhaps the most analyzed film of film history, studied by critics and specialists from different schools. Its "triumphal" course, according to the director's most distinguished biographer (Aranda, 1969), is unmatched as compared to Buñuel's shorts and, in general, to most of the noncommercial films ever made. This short has been considered the avatar of American independent film (Renan, 1968), and the initiator of the surrealist model in commercial film (Masterman, 1970) and of modern cinema in general (Bobker, 1969). The list of enthusiasts could be much longer. According to Noël Burch (1981), *Un Chien andalou* is the first film capable of making aggression one of cinema's structural elements. Octavio Paz (1951) considered it, together with *The Age of Gold*, as exemplary of the interconnectedness between film and poetry; for Charles Pornon (1959) it was the text that marked the transformation of the fantastic into the purely marvelous, and Alessandro Cappabianca (1972) regarded it, together with Cocteau's work, as the moment in which antirealism begins in cinema.

The evident, albeit unintentional, implication of such statements—even when accepted at their face value—is that of a mystification/recuperation of Buñuel's first work. Phillip Drummond (1977) was aware of this when he analyzed the film's opening sequence and the segment of the two pianos in one of the few textual analyses that have been made of the film.

As Dudley Andrew (1983) remarked:

> The institution of film proceeds not by the routine application of rules but by a tension between rules and a force of discourse trying to say something. This force overdetermines a sign within a conventional context so that the sign overflows both recognition and narrative placement, disturbing the system through misrecognition until, in the tension, we recognize what was meant. Such misrecognition can occur in the presentation of the

elementary cinematic sign, in its placement in a scene, in the scene's placement in the narrative and in the film's relation to a cultural context.

Referring to Andrew's text, Paul Sandro (1987) noted that while such an
evolutionist model might seem to grant Buñuel's films the power to change
the institution of cinema and the spectators' mentality, what it really accom-
plishes is an assessment of the limitations that confront all attempts at radical
change. If the model Andrew proposes implies that the discursive form of a
film like *Un Chien andalou* might correspond to a questioning of the drive
to interpretation, it is undoubtedly rather curious that the institution
responded by reducing the subversiveness of Buñuel's proposal through a
proliferation of interpretations. In this sense it is not gratuitous that the apparent "acceptance" on the part of the film industry at large of the director's
strategies once they were defined as surrealist and fixed as "artistic" models
worth imitating, meant indeed their "normalization" through the repeated
inclusion of dream sequences or similar effects in later narrative cinema.

Un Chien andalou has thus been turned into a sort of canonical model for
a difference that is not assumed as source for subversiveness, but is included
in the list of famous deviations, as an instance (even though a genial and
paradigmatic one) of the dysfunctions that necessarily go with a norm—
Hollywood narrative model—that is never really questioned as such.
Buñuel's *opera prima* can, from this perspective, be literally "worshiped" as
a specific historical phenomenon while erasing the radicality of its implications.

History of a Film Production

A complete history of the production process of *Un Chien andalou* is still to
come, but an outline can be attempted here, albeit summarily, by making use
of the data collected especially by José Francisco Aranda (1969), Salvador
Dalí (1942), Georges Sadoul (1965), and Randall Conrad (1976), among
others.

The film's project must be situated in the context of the relationship established by Buñuel and Dalí with the Paris avant-garde of the late 1920s. Although Dalí did not move to Paris until the beginning of 1929—the year *Un
Chien andalou* was made—the film represented the culmination of Buñuel's
long-standing relationship with vanguard cinema. Buñuel, who was six years

older than Dalí, had arrived in Paris in January 1925, one year after graduating from Madrid University with a degree in the humanities. In Paris he became part of the International Institute for Intellectual Cooperation, created in 1924 as the cultural branch of the League of Nations, where he worked as D'Ors's secretary. After a year he became actively involved in cinema and theater. Thanks to a recommendation from Pedro de Azcárate, who later became Spain's ambassador in London, Buñuel met pianist Ricardo Viñes, who got him the job that would be of crucial importance for his future.

One of Amsterdam's orchestras had performed very successfully Ramuz-Stravinsky's *History of a Soldier*, and the rival orchestra that Mengelberg directed, wanting to reply with something as remarkable, chose to perform one of Manuel de Falla's works. The viscountess of Noailles, who would later produce *The Age of Gold* with her husband, offered the Spanish composer her mansion for the rehearsals and the premiere of *Master Peter's Puppet Show*, commissioned by Winnaretta Singer. The orchestral version had made its debut in Seville in March 1921; the opera version was presented in Paris in June 1921. Having found out about the Amsterdam project from Mengelberg himself, Ricardo Viñes informed his cousin Hernando, who lived in Paris and was a close friend of Buñuel. The future director was asked to be in charge of the artistic direction of the opera's Dutch debut, which was to take place in Amsterdam on April 26, 1926. Buñuel moved to the Netherlands "without giving it even a thought," as he remembered years later in his conversations with Max Aub (1985), after rehearsing for fifteen days at Hernando Viñes's place. Buñuel described the production in his autobiography:

> The *retablo* refers to a small puppet theatre, and all the characters are
> marionettes whose voices are provided by the singers. I introduced some
> new twists by adding four real characters to the puppets; they were
> masked, and their role was to attend the puppeteer's, Maese Pedro's, per-
> formance and interrupt from time to time. Their voices too were provided
> by singers hidden in the orchestra pit. Of course, I got my friends to play
> the silent parts of the four people in the audience, which is how the cast
> came to include Cossio, Peinado (who played the innkeeper), and my cous-
> in Rafael Saura (Don Quixote). (Buñuel, 1984, 86–87)

The performance brought Buñuel fame and considerable success, certainly due in part to the presence in the cast of one of Europe's most celebrated opera singers of the time, Vera Janocópulos.

Buñuel's interest in scenography led him to enroll in the Paris Film Academy, directed by Camille Bardoux, Alex Allain, and Jean Epstein. He was Epstein's assistant director in two films, *Mauprat* (1926), where he also worked as an extra, and *The Fall of the House of Usher* (1928). Buñuel's collaboration with Epstein also includes his work in Mario Nalpas's and Henri Etiévant's *The Siren of the Tropics* (1927), whose main character was played by a young actress-dancer named Josephine Baker. During the shooting of this film Buñuel met actor Pierre Batcheff, actress Simone Mareuil, and cameraman Albert Dubergen, all of whom would later work on *Un Chien andalou*. Buñuel's assignment as assistant director ended when he refused to work with Abel Gance in *Napoleon* — which I personally consider the pseudomasterpiece of an overrated and megalomaniacal artisan. Buñuel would speak contemptuously of Gance on the occasion of the film's premiere:[1]

> I had my own ideas and taste about cinema. We were in the studios at Epinal and had planned to go out the next day to shoot the exteriors. Epstein told me: "Buñuel, Abel Gance will soon be here to try out and perhaps you could stay and give him a hand." I replied: "If it is Gance, I don't think I'm interested." "What are you talking about?" "I hate that kind of cinema." He told me: "*Qu'un petit con comme vous ose parler comme ça d'un homme aussi grand que Gance . . .* " [How can a little asshole like you dare to talk that way about a great director like Gance]. And added: "We are through, Buñuel; I'll drive you back to Paris if you wish." On the way to Paris he kept on giving me advice: "You seem rather surrealist. Beware of surrealists, they are crazy people." (Colina and Pérez Turrent, 1980: 20)

Buñuel made similar remarks to Max Aub (1985):

> He [Epstein] told me that I was to work with Abel Gance the next day; I told him I wouldn't work with a director I considered a very bad one. He became livid. "*Comment un petit con comme vous ose parle[r] ainsi d'un si grand metteur en scène!*" He later offered me a ride to Paris, though, for we were shooting in Epinal. (57)

Besides working as set decorator and assistant director, Buñuel was also a film critic for *La Gaceta Literaria Hispanoamericana* (end of 1927) and for *Les Cahiers d'Art* (March 1928). He wrote film reviews as well as articles of general interest, including some texts of relevance to our study, for they foreshadow some of his theoretical preoccupations about the cinematic medium; among these writings are "Del frame fotogénico" and "*Découpage* o segmentación cinegráfica," later collected by Sánchez-Vidal (1982). Buñuel's relentless activism as critic and cultural agitator did not prevent him from working on two subsequent projects: one was about Goya, for Julio César's company, and the other was supposed to be his first film, *Los caprichos*, a story in six scenes whose script he was writing in collaboration with Ramon Gómez de la Serna. It is not clear what happened to these two projects, although it is certain that the funding intended for *Los caprichos* was used to write, shoot, and edit *Un Chien andalou* during the first three months of 1929. The film was shown at the Studio Ursulines in April, according to the information provided by Cyril Connolly (quoted in Drummond, 1977), before its public screening at Studio 28 in the fall.

It was important, however, that in the case of the former project a decision was made to pay a tribute to Goya. In fact, 1927 was the year in which Góngora's centennial was celebrated. The anniversary served not only to revive the work by the poet from Córdoba, but also and perhaps especially to institutionalize, under the poet's name, some artistic and discursive standpoints that were incompatible with the views of the most radical writers and intellectuals of the time. Goya's centennial (he had died in 1828) could be used equally well to claim this alternative posture. It was not by chance that Valle-Inclán was, together with Buñuel and Gómez de la Serna, among the proponents of this group; his *Tirano Banderas* (1927) and "esperpentos" were unmistakable evidence of his determination to offer alternatives to an artistic practice that was eventually to be too easily assimilated by dominant discourse. Agustín Sánchez-Vidal (1988) has discussed the way in which the publicity regarding Góngora's centennial implied a silence about Goya's, with the attendant silencing of the proposals that Goya's work implied: the introduction of "expressionist modes, the influence of Quevedo and of the 'esperpentos,' and the bases for the subsequent neo-romantic and surrealist developments." This can perhaps explain the meaning of the title *Un Chien andalou*, as testimony of the attack against a certain understanding of aesthetics prompted fundamentally by Andalusian artists and writers—not only García Lorca—from radical political and ideological standpoints. That the analysis of the Gongorean celebration as a major cultural and political strategy is more than a tendentious interpretation is demonstrated by the fact that, from a different angle and single-handedly, but with the same will to propose an alternative, Luis Cernuda chose the Garcilaso model for his *Egloga, elegía, oda* at about the same time (Talens, 1975).

Valle-Inclán, who had defined Góngora as "unbearable" in June 1927 in *La Gaceta Literaria*, was one of the few members of the older generation to understand the importance of the new medium.[2] He had also thought of making a film on Goya. Buñuel found out about his project from García Lorca and went to see him. Valle-Inclán gave up the idea of making the film, but not without telling Buñuel, with his well-known irony, as Sánchez-Vidal (1988) recounts: "I believe you will make a much better film than I would, because you are a professional, but please do not forget to point out that Goya became deaf when he repaired the axle of the Duchess of Alba's coach."

Gómez de la Serna was replaced by Salvador Dalí, whom Buñuel had met at the time of the Residencia de Estudiantes in Madrid. The director-to-be's original idea—initially called *El mundo por diez céntimos*, later *Los caprichos*—was rejected apparently because of Dalí's distaste for its naive sentimentality. There may have been other reasons that motivated the decision to forsake the project. In Aub (1985), Santiago Ontañón has noted that

> at first [Buñuel] had wanted to make a film about life in a newspaper. . . .
> Then he saw . . . *Rien que les heures* . . . and that changed the whole
> thing. Well, that was his idea, really. This made him change his mind,
> since it may have smacked of plagiarism to go on with his original project.
> That's when he decided he wanted to do *Goya*. . . . He was obsessed
> with Goya. (318)

Between January and mid-February 1929 the two friends began working on a script in Figueras. It was first called *El Marista en la ballesta*, then successively *Défense de se pencher dehors* and *Défense de se pencher dedans*. Later Dalí proposed to use for the film the title of an early collection of poems by Buñuel, *Un Chien andalou* (An Andalusian dog).

The collaborative work between Dalí and Buñuel on the literary script has been one of the most unsettling elements in the critical approach to the film as finished product. In some of the studies most explicitly centered on a hermeneutical reading of the final result, in effect both phases of the production process of *Un Chien andalou*—the writing of the literary script and the actual shooting—are considered equivalent. In Cesarman (1976), for example, the chapter that deals with *Un Chien andalou* (leaving aside the reductionism of the analytical approach adopted by the author, which is the product of a mechanical application of Freudian psychoanalysis)[3] includes detailed explications of the meaning of elements that do not even appear in the film: the violence of the rain in the second sequence, the inner silent music that the androgyne listens to, the presence of the lame man in the middle segment, and so on.

Leaving aside Buñuel's explicit statements about his authorship of the finished product (Dalí was present during only one session of the shooting), the mechanisms of both textual spaces cannot be confused. The "automaticity"—let us call it that for the moment—of the literary script has nothing to do with the precision and rationality that characterize the editing of the finished film. Between the two moments exists the abyss that separates the postulates of the surrealist avant-garde (typical of the Catalan painter) from those of a practice that would be more adequately defined in terms of radical realism. As we shall attempt to demonstrate, Buñuel's statements about his total adherence to surrealist principles in *La Révolution Surréaliste* (see appendix 1)—apart from the fact that they introduce the script, not the film—should be understood as what they really were: a public confession of orthodoxy forced by the movement's Sovereign Pontiff, rather than a declaration of aesthetic or moral principles. In any case, explicative texts so close to the genre "manifesto" cannot supplant what a detailed analysis of the textual space unmistakably reveals. We shall return to this issue.

Closer to the film's real structure is the second statement about the definition of *Un Chien andalou* as a "desperate, passionate call to crime." What Buñuel underscores in fact is that the film does not narrate a dream, but takes advantage of mechanisms analogous to those of dreams; that is, he does not mix up the properties of the raw material with those belonging to the work performed on it. The consequences of this proposal are, in my opinion, quite evident. The idea is that of (a) operating on the perceptual devices irrationally assumed by the common spectator; and (b) staging the arbitrariness of a too easy and too often unquestioned symbolism. In this sense *Un Chien andalou* is not, and does not pretend to be, a "vanguardist" film; it is, rather, quite the opposite. Buñuel's film reinscribes the history of the cinema at the time of its making. Its deliberate "antiartistic" imprint can be viewed therefore as a virulent reaction to the vanguard cinema of the time (which Buñuel regarded as addressing exclusively the spectator's reason and artistic sensibility) with its play of light and shadow, its photographic effects, its preoccupation with rhythmic editing and search for new technical procedures—all this accomplished in a perfectly reasonable and conventional way.

Un Chien andalou questions the notion of the "new" that ultimately seemed to ground the historical practice of the avant-gardes by operating dialectically on the conventional processes of spectatorial identification and by bringing about in such practice instinctive reactions of attraction/repulsion. There is nothing in fact more distant from *The Seashell and the Clergyman* or *Entr'acte* than *Un Chien andalou*.[4] Actor Pierre Batcheff's presence in the film—the prototype of the young beau of the French cinema of the 1920s—in a role that refers back to the one Buñuel played in *The Siren of the Tropics*, should be read in this sense.

In Man Ray's *L'étoile de mer*, for example, based on a poem by Robert Desnos, there is an explicit intention to narrativize the suggestions of poetic discourse. To a certain extent, the film can be read as the transformation of the poem's images into argumental structure. The same narrative logic also pervades, to quote another example of "vanguardist" cinema, René Clair's *Paris qui dort*, where the new perspective on the real that the new medium allowed (freeze frame, and so on) is assumed by the narrative itself and reduced to an explication by the narrative's argumental logic: everything is the effect of a ray that a scientist is experimenting with. Buñuel, who acknowledged the influence of Benjamin Péret on *Un Chien andalou*, approaches the issue in a different fashion.

> I had already become interested in the surrealists, without really knowing any of them; among them, I was especially interested in Benjamin Péret. I saw him for the first time in this film. I was never interested in him as a person, but his poems really struck me. Later, while I was making *Un Chien andalou*, his poems came often to my mind. (Aub, 1985, 57)

This reference is not noticeable in the film because Buñuel, unlike Man Ray, does not take the anecdotal support from poetic discourse and does not attempt to translate the suggestiveness of its images. Instead, he is interested in applying to narrative the compositional mechanisms proper to poetic discourse.

The film's script was published for the first time in the final issue of *La Révolution Surréaliste* in December 1929. The funding for the film came from the 25,000 pesetas that Buñuel's mother had decided to contribute to his previous project, *Los caprichos*. We know nothing of the film's editing phase, although Buñuel declared that all the effects were made with the camera during the shooting and not later in the lab (although it is hard to believe this about some specific cases, such as frame 215). Credit is given to only two actors, Pierre Batcheff and Simone Mareuil (as a matter of fact the film plays with variants of the two characters that Batcheff and Mareuil play), although there were other people in bit parts, among them Buñuel himself, the actor playing the young man at the beach, and Dalí and Catalan anarchist Jaime Miravilles, who played the roles of the two Marist brothers (as the découpage of the film shows, a third actor substituted for Dalí in one of these shots). From a technical point of view the only one to be credited is the director of photography, Duverger (Albert Dubergen), even though it seems that set decorator Pierre Schilzneck's contribution to the production design was also rather conspicuous. The extras for the scenes on the street and in the meadow were chosen during the shooting from among the customers of a nearby coffee shop.

The history of the production of *Un Chien andalou* does not end here. In 1960 the film acquired a new textual status with the addition of a sound track under the supervision of Buñuel. The decision to add a sound track had been made by Raymond Rohauer, curator of Les Grands Films Classiques, in an attempt to renew the film's copyright and reproduce the phonograph music that had accompanied its opening in 1929.

The Structure of the Film

The problems following the film's opening as well as the scandal surrounding its reception are part of film history's collection of anecdotes. Let us now turn to a closer analysis of the film itself.

The story that *Un Chien andalou* seems to narrate centers on the relationship between a man and a woman: in order of appearance, Pierre Batcheff and Simone Mareuil. As neither of the characters has a name, we shall therefore call them "man" and "woman." The way their story is narrated does not allow an approach to the film in accordance with the classical analytical model. The film's continuous rupture of the logic of the events and of the relationship between sequences, the eccentricity with which spaces superimpose and merge while apparently keeping all the *raccords* of editing (at least as many as possible), the constant mixing of the different points of view with a logic that is, as we shall see, ultimately implacable, set this text apart from both the conventions of the classical narrative model and the gratuitous abstraction of the contemporary cinematic avant-gardes.

To make our reading easier, let us briefly examine the order of the events as they develop in the film.[5]

After the opening credits, a black screen appears bearing the inscription *Once upon a time* . . . A man sharpens a razor by a window. When he is done, he steps out onto a balcony. A white cloud is moving toward the full moon. Intercut of a man's hand holding by a woman's eye the same razor we saw being sharpened; she sits in the foreground facing the camera. After a shot of a thin cloud passing across the full moon, the razor cuts an eye in extreme close-up; a viscous fluid oozes out of the eye onto its lower lid.

Another black screen bears the inscription *Eight years later*. A young man is riding a bicycle on a deserted street. He wears white frilly cuffs, a cap with white wings, a collar, and a frilly skirt over his dark suit, similar to those accessories adorning little girls' dresses, but also recalling the white-and-blue striped dusters worn by the students at the Marist brothers' schools. A woman — apparently the same that had her eye slit a moment before — sits in the middle of a room, looking attentively at a book. The man on the bicycle loses his balance and falls astride his bicycle onto the sidewalk. The woman seems to anticipate the fall; she lifts her head in sudden amazement and listens for something, then goes to the window (a window similar to the one we saw before, next to which the man was sharpening the razor in the opening sequence) leans forward, and sees the man. She rushes down the stairs and out to the street, kneels by the fallen man, and kisses him passionately; then she picks up the small box that the man had carried, hanging from his neck.

A dissolve shows the woman back in her room as she opens the box, which contains a necktie with diagonal stripes and a white collar. The woman places both items next to the frilly cuffs, cap, and skirt on the bedspread, then sits and stares at them with an odd look. She seems to become aware of someone's presence behind her. When she turns, the cyclist in his dark suit — without the frilly cuffs, cap, skirt, and necktie — is standing at the other side of the room staring at his right hand. The woman stands up and walks toward him. Big live ants in the palm of his hand seem to come out of a dark hole in the middle of his palm. The shot of the crawling ants dissolves successively into a close-up of a woman's armpit, a sea urchin, and a young woman in a crowd who is poking with a stick at a severed hand lying in the street. From the window above, the man and the woman look at what is happening in the street. A policeman picks up the severed hand, places it in a striped box identical to the one the cyclist carried, and gives it to the young woman. As cars speed around her, the young woman, clasping the box, seems to be unable to move. She is eventually run down by a car and lies on the ground, with the box by her side.

In the room the man, seemingly excited from the scene he has just witnessed, tries to seduce the woman. His hands stroke her breasts through her dress. The woman pushes him away, then scrambles over the bed and takes shelter behind a chair in a corner. He seems to be at a loss, and looks for something on the floor. He bends to pick up two ends of rope, then straightens up, tugging at the ropes; his mysterious cargo seems to prevent him from moving forward. A shot from behind shows his load: two grand pianos with two dead donkeys and two Marist brothers on top. Terrified, the woman makes a dash for the door at her side. The man lets go of the ropes and tries to follow her, but the door closes behind her and traps his hand. Another shot shows his hand crawling with ants. The woman turns, pushing the door shut on his hand—we are back in the room she has just left—and sees the cyclist lying on the bed, wearing the cap, the skirt, and the striped necktie.

Another black screen bears the inscription *About 3 A.M.* A man wearing a hat and seen from behind rings a doorbell. The woman crosses the room to open the door; she will remain off scene during all of the following sequence. The stranger orders the man lying in bed to get up, strips him of the white frills he is wearing, and throws them out the window. Then he has him stand against the wall, raise his arms, and stretch them against the wall.

Another black screen bears the inscription *Sixteen years before.* The stranger walks toward the camera. His face is the same as the other man's. He moves toward a school desk, picks up a book and a notebook, and gives them to the man standing against the wall. The two objects suddenly become revolvers; the man prepares to shoot the stranger. With a merciless, sadistic expression, he finally fires.

The wounded man falls in a different space: a park in the script, a meadow with a lake in the distance in the film. He tries to hold on to the naked back of a woman whose profile is very similar to that of the woman in the room, but her body fades before he reaches the ground. Several people walk quickly toward the stricken man lying on the grass and, when they realize he is dead, they look for someone with the authority to decide what to do; at this person's command, they pick up the body and carry it as in a funeral. Fade out to the room, as the woman opens the door to go in.

A moth appears on the screen, with a death's-head pattern on its back. The man with the revolvers is in the room again, with a pensive expression on his face. He suddenly claps his hand to his mouth; when he removes it, his mouth has disappeared. Hairs—thick, short hairs, like those from an armpit—grow now in the place where the mouth used to be. When the woman sees this she looks concerned and touches her armpit only to realize that her armpit has no hairs at all. Evidently irritated, she reacts by applying lipstick to her lips; then she puts a shawl on her shoulders and exits through the same door she came in. This time, however, she exits to a beach where another young man awaits her. The young man seems to resent her being late; she strokes him tenderly and kisses him. The two walk away holding each other as they stroll along the stony shore, where the cuffs, the collar, the skirt, the box, and the strap that we saw thrown out of the window all lie. One more black screen says *In spring* . . . over the man and the woman buried up to their chests in sand at the deserted beach. Fade out.

The first thing to note after this brief summary is that the film's content and development are very far from resembling what one traditionally expects from a narrative that begins so explicitly with *Once upon a time* . . . The surprise increases when we realize that the same character—the man Pierre Batcheff portrays—also plays the roles of three other characters: the cyclist, the man whose hand crawls with ants, and the "double" murdered by the latter. All these figures coexist, located as they are simultaneously in mutually exclusive spaces. This character seems endowed with magical powers: he enters the woman's room (without anyone having opened the door) only a few moments after we saw him lie motionless and wounded on the sidewalk; he has ants crawl out of his hand; he carries pianos, dead donkeys, and Marist brothers into the room where most of the action seems to take place; he has his hand trapped in the door while being able to walk across the room, finally to appear lying peacefully in bed; he transforms school objects into deadly weapons; he can erase his mouth and have a woman's armpit hairs appear in its place. Another series of events disseminated in the film produces the same sort of disconcertedness: the woman's eye that we saw being slit in the sequence/prologue seems to be in perfect condition eight years later; the young woman that is run over by a car is in possession of the box we know to be placed on the bed in the woman's bedroom; the walk along the beach at the end of the film turns into an inexplicable burial in which the young man accompanying the woman is replaced by the main male character. We witness, moreover, a constant disruption of the narrative logic whose syntactic order is nonetheless scrupulously respected. The hand with crawling ants suddenly appears, severed, in the middle of the street; the "double" murdered in the room falls in a totally different space; when the characters go out the door, they enter a place identical to the one they have just left, or they reach an improbable beach bordering the third floor of the building where the action is supposed to take place. Finally, the sound track alternates tango music and music by Wagner in a contradictory way, breaking the merely descriptive function assigned it by the classical syntax.

All this does not prevent the film from having a seemingly ironlike narrative structure, intercut with the intertitles that Michel Marie (1977) considers to be a parody of those used in the silent classical cinema as they show the freezing effect of a certain type of rhetorical scansion of temporal durations.

Such structure consists of the narration of a more or less coherent story with a beginning, a development, and an end in a process that is logical or verisimilar to different degrees.

The story following the initial *Once upon a time* . . . corresponds to the fulfilling of the expectations raised by storytelling, that is to say, it is the mise-en-scène of a presence that affirms both its intention to narrate a story and its power over the elements by means of which—and about which—it narrates. This is what happens in the first sequence with the shocking shot of the slit eye, as we soon shall see. What is shown is the apparently arbitrary logic of the "cut and paste" that produces as a rhetorical effect a continuity between shots that the shots by themselves do not have if analyzed individually.

This presence has a double function and justifies the accumulative and fragmentary character of the sequences as well as their interconnectedness, thus making of the work as a whole a sort of fragmentary body. It is certainly not by chance that the words "Un Chien andalou" limit themselves to *name*, rather than *title*, the object. There are no dogs in the film, nor are there Andalusians. This has led some critics, such as Aranda (1969) and Sánchez-Vidal (1988), to interpret *Un Chien andalou* as a veiled attack by Buñuel on his contemporary writers and, more specifically, as an attack on Federico García Lorca.

> Buñuel, Dalí, Bello and other friends from the North [of Spain] called *Andalusian dogs* the Andalusians at the Residencia de Estudiantes, poets who were insensitive to the revolutionary poetry of social content that Buñuel envisaged perhaps before anyone else in Spain (Alberti and others would follow this path years later). If we think of this we shall realize indeed that *Un Chien andalou* describes a sort of biographical trajectory that—in its subconscious and proto-paranoic facet—is applicable to many in the group: it describes their infantilism, castration complex, sexual ambivalence, identity problems, etc., and their inner struggle to get rid of their bourgeois heritage to let the adult person free. (Aranda, 1976, 46)

Buñuel always denied such an interpretation of the film's title. In an interview with José de la Colina and Tomás Pérez Turrent published in *Contracampo*, he stated the following:

> That's not the way it is. People find allusions wherever they want to. Federico García Lorca and I were angry at each other for some time. When I was in New York in the thirties, Angel del Río told me that, when he visited him, Federico had said: "Buñuel has made a tiny piece of shit called *Un Chien andalou*, and I am the Andalusian dog." It wasn't true at all. *Un Chien andalou* was the title of a collection of poems that I had written.

The anecdote is important because it underscores the difference between Buñuel and the other writers, such as García Lorca, who constituted the

Spanish avant-garde. These other writers considered the referential character of artistic discourse as ineludible and labeled as "antiartistic" a proposal,
like Buñuel's, that reached beyond the field of cinema and dealt with the
wider level of discourse in general. We shall return to this issue in chapter 3.

In this sense the film is not titled but rather called *Un Chien andalou*, in
the same way in which the director's name is Luis, or the actors' names are
Pierre and Simone. The name implies nothing but the trace of a power imposed on the object by whoever is granted the object's authorship. Coherently with what we defined before in terms of poetic discourse, Buñuel's film
does not impose meanings, it offers proposals for making sense. For the
name *is not integrated as title*, it *superimposes itself as a brand* of the ineludible presence of an agency external to the object and which cannot be identified with its speaking subject. This agency assumes social authorship by imposing a name that is not bound to maintain any relationship with the reality
of said object.

At the same time, the chronological anarchy, the false *raccords*, the jump
cuts (a rather frequent technique in the film practice of the time), as well as
the recurring presence of certain objects and bodily figures ambulating like
ghosts on the flat surface of the screen, acquire a sense—even though they
do not have a specific meaning—thanks to the relationship they establish
with each other or with other elements of the textual space that constitutes
and inscribes them. Thus the box with diagonal stripes says or suggests nothing by itself (indeed, Buñuel held little esteem for the reductive allegorical interpretations usually made of his films)[6] but only through its recurrence in
the filmic text. "No symbols where none intended," the Beckettian narrator
would say in *Watt*. Likewise, the actors' faces or bodies are nothing but neutral marks that refer to nothing and evoke nothing; that is, they do not signify
because they do not *represent*. Their relationship with other faces and bodies
within a frame or the film's overall textual space does not grant them meaning; instead, it turns them into elements capable of producing sense. *Thus
the film as a whole is not organized as a communicable meaning but as a proposal for possible senses.* This is possibly what constitutes the radical novelty
of Buñuel's work.

From this point of view and aware of the risk it implies, we can attempt
an approach to the complex problem of the film's structure by beginning with
the beginning. We can begin, that is, with a description of the sections that
distinctive marks of delimitation define as such in the textual space of the
film.

We can trace the existence of five big blocks separated by intertitles bearing information that is punctual and vague at the same time: punctual because it offers very concrete and specific data (once upon a time, eight years later, about 3 A.M., sixteen years before, in spring); vague because it is not at all clear to what such precision refers. These five parts coexist with another simultaneous distribution of the material in three big unities that are designated by taking as reference point not the existence of the five intertitles, but the presence or absence of certain elements. The first part (shots 1–12) is defined by the presence of the man with the razor and comprises the text's prologue. The second part (shots 13–289) centers its narrative lines on the two main characters, the man and the woman. Finally, shot 290—the film's only freeze frame—places us in the epilogue and constitutes the text's third and last part.

The second part can be divided in turn into four blocks made of two, four, four, and two segments respectively by taking as point of reference the closured actions that develop in these segments. The table included in appendix 3 contains and specifies such division in accordance with the distribution of frames in appendixes 1 and 2.

The Prologue as Contextualization

If we rely on the fact that we are going to be told a story (and this is what the initial intertitle is clearly meant to accomplish), the first surprising thing in the first segment, defined as the text's prologue, is the presence of a character (played by Luis Buñuel) that will then disappear for good from the film, physically in shot 9 and as effect of editing after shot 12. His presence is counterweighed by the absence from this sequence of the man who will later be the protagonist of the remainder of the film. This arbitrariness seems to raise questions about the function of the segment. Various possible senses, however, can be attributed to this segment in relation with the rest of the film. They can be summarized as pertaining to three different categories: (a) the cinematic fact; (b) the filmic discourse; and (c) *Un Chien andalou* as specific film.

With regard to the first category, it is obvious that what distinguishes the cinematic phenomenon from other traditional discursive manifestations susceptible to being included within the categories that we have defined as textual spaces of the first kind (see "Text vs. Textual Space" in chapter 1) is essentially the passivity cinema presupposes in the spectator at the moment of reception. A book, for example, is not read by itself. The reader has to make a physical effort, follow the trajectory of the printed characters on the page, compounding the words and then the sentences in order to follow the written text. In order for a painting to be perceived as such and not as a neutral element of a set, the viewer must voluntarily direct his or her gaze on the canvas surface, in order to be able to relate the colors and have access to the intelligibility of what the painting's composition proposes. In the case of cinema, no voluntary act is exacted other than going to a movie theater, buying a ticket at the box office, and sitting in a dark room: this is what constitutes the social act of "going to the movies." From that moment on, the spectator simply can let the images impregnate his or her retina in what we could define as a state of "nonattentive vision." The impossibility of the projected image's going backward (the use of the flatbed or of video copies is proper to scholars, specialists, or modern spectators; it does not belong to the average spectator's habits, and certainly was not part of the viewing experience during the first decades of this century) determines that the film can be literally injected in the spectator if she or he is not fully conscious and does not intervene actively in the act of reception. The first American filmmakers were aware of this. The historical construction of what Noël Burch, through the analysis of Porter's films, has defined as the "institutional mode of representation" (IMR) was founded on the assumption of this principle. To erase from the material the traces of its construction—the so-called invisible editing—was a way to contribute to spectatorial passivity. The spectator was in this way practically alienated from himself or herself in the images on the screen.

When Buñuel slits open the woman's eye with a razor in a close-up, the physical aggression suffered by the spectator's sleeping sensitivity prevents the viewer from continuing to look passively, if not motivating him or her to decide to leave the movie theater at once altogether. The mere conditioned reflex of preparing oneself for a new aggression physically forces the spectator to adopt an active attitude toward the screen.

Yet the series of shot / countershots establishing a connection between the man by the window and the white cloud passing across the face of the full moon stages—according to the logic of the institutional narrative editing—the spectator's point of view, inscribing it in the materiality of the screen. The subjective shot of *the man looking in the film* places him in the same position as *the spectator watching the film* in the dark of the movie theater. Indeed, they look at the same thing at the same time. The same process, although in the opposite direction, connects the spectator with the eye-slitting man as synecdochical effect of the hand holding the razor on the screen, creating for the spectator a position already integrated in the filmic discourse. It is not by chance that this displacement is explicitly underscored by the fact that the man holding the razor wears a necktie, whereas the character in the previous frames does not.[7] At the same time, the relationship of contiguity established through editing between the full moon and the woman's eye determines the identification of the woman's (and/or the moon's) position with that of the spectator. The spectator thus becomes the subject and the object of the action: someone looking at the slitting of an eye, someone whose eye is slit, and someone who symbolically slits an eye. This act, closured for being presented as such, nonetheless allows the elaboration of a sense, if we keep in mind that what we are watching is a film and that filmic discourse functions as a mechanism that has to do precisely with what we are watching on the screen. By blinding—*crossing out and branding*—the spectator's eye and substituting it with the (invisible) eye of the camera, a film determines not only what we watch but also at what time and from where. The filmic discourse never reproduces reality, it re/produces it as someone's interpretation inscribed as editing. The editing is therefore the real *speaking subject* of the filmic enunciation. The (false) notion of cinema as imitation of reality (cinema is life), which grounds the IMR, gives way to a more accurate understanding of cinema as exposition and objectivization of a specific point of view, individual or collective, articulated and inscribed by what we have defined in terms of editing/speaking subject. The difference between fictional and documentary form, and the concept of authorship as pertaining to an individualized psychological entity appear not to be pertinent issues at all, as I have pointed out in a different context (Talens, 1985, 1987).

A first sense can be attributed to this violent and apparently gratuitous opening sequence: that of exposing the procedure by which the story about to develop on the screen is being told. It is quite interesting that Buñuel himself—the film's director and author (editor)—plays the part of the man slitting the eye, thus assuming the double function as spectator and performer of the event. Even if he is not entirely in the frame in the segment's most revealing frames, he is inscribed synecdochically: the razor assumes his function. Buñuel the author gives way to Buñuel-apparatus, that is, Buñuel as authorial machinery.[8]

Author and spectator carry out complementary roles. The man slitting the eye (presumably the woman's eye, as the editing leads one to believe) not only stages the narrative procedure of the film, but also originates a story that will somehow have to do with eye-slitting. The woman in this first segment-prologue is the same woman who will appear in the rest of the film, a film that, as we shall see, alludes to voyeurism and erotic sublimation.

We already have, then, in principle, at least three different directions of/for sense proposed by the prologue to the spectator; they are not signified directly by the prologue itself, but are the result of the relationships established with the categories previously mentioned. The prologue constitutes a mapping of the mechanisms underlying both cinematic practice and filmic discourse while introducing a point of view that allows the spectator to articulate coherently the fragments that comprise the film as a whole. By acting actively on the former aspect, the latter one allows in turn the establishment of a relationship not only with this film but with cinema as such — as discourse — and the voyeurism of everyday life. Not in vain does each film inscribed in the narrative mode of representation locate the spectator in the privileged position of the voyeur who sees without being seen (Cavell, 1971). For this reason, as Juan-Miguel Company (1978) wrote, the discourse of cinema is, by definition, pornographic in the widest sense of the word, that is, producer of reality effects for spectators/voyeurs. Because of this, the so-called pornographic cinema is the kind of cinema that best defines, by reduction to the absurd, the basic procedures proper of filmic discourse.[9]

But there's more than that. If Buñuel is the story's narrator, the slitting of the eye is also showing us the necessity to cross out the conventional gaze with which we look at cinema — and reality — in order to be able (a) to watch his film with innocent, nonmanipulated eyes; and (b) to look at reality (on which we found our interpretive categories, whether consciously or unconsciously) with new eyes. This is how we shall be able to accomplish Lautréamont's proposal to "discover beauty in the least expected encounter: on a dissecting table, a sewing machine, or an umbrella."

By complying with narrative logic, however, this cut turns the viewer into a listener (see note 8 of this chapter). If voyeurism is associated to the primal scene, the child's desire to see the parents' sexual intercourse, and if this act of watching is in turn associated to the child's listening to the sounds generated during the sexual act, it would seem coherent to introduce in the field of vision a substitution of the descriptive role of music of traditional sound tracks with noise, understood both in the broad and in the semiotic sense of the word. In most of Buñuel's later films this displacement is even more evident than in *Un Chien andalou*.

In effect this is what Ducasse expressed with his question "These eyes are not yours; where did you get them from?" The capability to discover the unusual goes hand in hand with the possibility to deconstruct the normal logic of the gaze. The collage technique, so typical in *Un Chien andalou* and so often used by Buñuel in his later films, demands this deconstruction. Carlos Fuentes (1976) defined this very well when he stated:

> The object, the face, the foot, or the gesture, chosen from an abundant and nearly immobile disorder, acquires an unbearable relief; they are revealed in a previously unthinkable connection with a totality in which Buñuel plunges us again at once, without lingering to celebrate the lyricalness of the moment.

In short, Buñuel forces us to "perceive" differently. To interpret this segment in terms of an allegory of birth from the moment of conception (the sharpening of the razor) to the trauma of birth (the slitting of the eye), through the process of the fetus's growth (the full moon), as Mondragon (1949) proposes, or as an allegory of the post- rather than prenatal phase (Durgnat, 1967), is only the product of a decontextualization of an ensemble of shots. Such interpretation grants these shots symbolic status per se, without analyzing the reasons why they are placed where they are in the overall textual space of the film.

Linda Williams's (1981) approach is, from this point of view, much more adequate and interesting. She reads the prologue as a sort of metaphor of "surrealist cinema" because of the use of a rare type of filmic figure that she defines, following Christian Metz, as "metaphor placed in syntagm." Such figure is characterized by a reversal of the ordering of the relationship between the elements of reality and those of the metaphorical level.

Williams's reflections are an important point of reference. She divides the initial segment in three units: (a) shots 1 to 4; (b) shots 5 to 7; and (c) shots 8 to 12. The apparent logic of a supposedly narrative editing would lead us to associate, for example, shots 1 and 3 with shots 2 and 4, in spite of the very subtle yet notable differences: the window in shots 1 and 3 does not have shades, which do appear in shots 2 and 4; the displacement of the camera in shots 2 and 4 from the position it occupied in shots 1 and 3 maintains the *raccord* of the axis. (It is not so, however, with the figure on the screen, whose left side is turned toward the window in shots 1 and 3, and in the opposite direction in shots 2 and 4.) This series of shots/countershots—after shots 5 and 7, in medium shot, which reinforce the spectator's illusion that a spatial relationship exists between shots 1 and 3 and shots 2 and 4— anticipates the series that organizes the third unit, though with an important reversal. In the first unit the order is "seen object + man's gaze." In the third unit we have the opposite: "gaze + seen object" (the full moon), which also implies a reversal of the causal relationship between the elements.

Leaving aside Williams's considerations about the alternating of distinct, equivalent spaces through editing, it is important to underscore a first and significant consequence deriving from her analysis: the causal relationship gaze/object becomes the causal relationship gaze/event and constitutes the main device by which to understand the film's overall development.

Phillip Drummond (1977), who values negatively a first version of the aforementioned analysis while acknowledging the pertinence of the description on which it is based, sustains that the prologue cannot be considered an anticipation of the rest of the film. He argues on the basis of the various displacements and changes in perspective and setting that the film presents and because of the impossibility to locate realistically the space where the characters are situated. (He states, for example, that one cannot be certain that the woman is seated on the balcony when her eye is slit, as Williams suggests; I believe, on the contrary, that one can be positive about it, although this is a marginal question in the present argument.) According to Drummond the window we see in this fragment is not the same as the one we see later; likewise he thinks that the room where the action is set later in the film is different from the room we see at the beginning of the film. These remarks are based, from my point of view, on the need to submit the discourse of *Un Chien andalou* to a narrative logic that is diegetically classical, when this is clearly not appropriate for this film.

First of all, the film's later development does not show one window, but two: one in the segment of the severed hand, the other in the segment of the "double." Second, what differentiates the two spaces is less the presence/absence of certain fixed descriptive features than the different positioning of the camera (even though the lack of plants in the segment of the "double," for example, can be justified from a narrative point of view by keeping in mind that the action develops eight and sixteen years before, respectively).

The camera is located at the level of the window in the prologue segment, and at street level in the central block, so that in the latter case the window is seen in a low angle shot. The law of verisimilitude is respected here, yet not in the opening segment, where no internal reason seems to justify the positioning of the camera in an impossible place, up in the air. Interestingly enough, this break in the sequence's verisimilitude, shown so explicitly, appears in the segment where the narrator lays open the rules of the game. Nothing indicates that the room is not the same, and nothing indicates the opposite either; in the opening segment we see the window with shades and curtains, and they are at least quite similar to the ones that we see, in long shot, hanging from the window in the middle part of the film. According to the classical logic that Drummond implicitly seems to claim, a character cannot enter the frame from the right immediately after exiting it through the left. A break in the continuity breaks the spectator's spatial reference points, and is confusing. In *Un Chien andalou*, however, these principles are rigorously respected, even though with enough transgressions to devoid them of specific meaning. The aim is not to "mislead" the spectator, but to force him or her to take a stand whose values have not been established definitively beforehand. The dissolves, for example, have the function they are supposed to have: they are marks of transition (as with shots 251 and 252, and 283 and 284). Yet their classical function at a spatial and temporal level is at times mixed together with a merely syntactical function, to connect signifiers, which preempts their normative function. This happens, for example, in shots 58 to 61, and 253 to 258.

Because of its paradigmatic character, such procedure should not be disregarded, especially considering that this is the only instance of transgression or inversion to exist from the film's very beginning, at the moment when the credits appear on the screen. In the credits only two intertitles are connected to one another by means of a direct cut: the one bearing the words "*Un Chien andalou*" (photogram 1) and the one with the name of the director (photogram 2). All the other credits (photograms 3 to 7) are connected by means of dissolves. It is as though the film's physical beginning itself makes explicit that one element of the film's overall structure subsumes and articulates all the other elements of the text.

That the supposed main character disappears from the film after shot 12, or that the woman whose eye was slit appears eight years later with her eyes intact, may in effect simply indicate, as Drummond remarked, that the function of this segment is merely to "satisfy the rites of narrative exposition" (103): to inscribe a principle, so that there is one, and move on to something else, with no consequences whatsoever. However, an analytical avenue can be pointed out that does not take for granted that what we really see after this segment is the story of the relationship between a man and a woman; rather, this analysis would seem to suggest that we are watching the story that one single character—the woman—hallucinates or remembers in the course of the film.

It seems that the image of the woman's face displaces, redefines, and eventually ejects from the film the presence of the "man-author," a process that Noël Burch and Jorge Dana (1974), writing about *The Cabinet of Dr. Caligari*, defined as the "expulsion and / or radical questioning of the orientation codes . . . through a strategical return to frontality." This does not

imply that her face is, as Drummond remarks, the instigator of the man's violence in the sequence of the two pianos, a sequence metaphorically connected
to the full moon that the man can relate to only as voyeur — first, because
what triggers his violence (his desire) derives, through editing, from the
shared, albeit differently assumed, viewing of the young woman as she is run
over by a car, and second, because it presupposes to connect the man with
the razor (Buñuel) with the protagonist of the rest of the film (Batcheff)
through a series of identifications that the film does not allow us to perform
if we abide strictly to the materiality of the text.

The Central Block: The Narrative Anecdote as
Projection of the Woman's Gaze

Much more complex than the issues arising from an analysis of the prologue
are the questions posed by a viewing of the 277 shots that follow. Let us examine them thoroughly.

If we keep in mind what we noted earlier about Linda Williams's work,
we will notice something quite interesting and peculiar in the complex compositional structure of *Un Chien andalou*: the syntagmatic relationship established between shots by the editing seems to create a direct, almost causal
relationship between the events and the characters' gazes. The man looks at
his hand (shot 50), and we see ants crawling on the palm of his hand (shot
51); he watches with undisguised anxiety as the young woman is run over
by a car (shot 100), and the sequence of the seduction or rape attempt begins
immediately after (shots 101ff.); he looks down at something lying on the
floor offscreen (shot 133), and two pianos hanging from ropes appear, followed by the Marist brothers and the dead donkeys (shots 134ff.), and so on.

The same happens with the woman. She stares with a somewhat concen-
trated anxiety in the direction of the camera (shots 45 and 47), and the necktie lying on the bedspread ties itself around the collar (shots 46 and 48); at
the end of this sequence she turns her eyes toward the other end of the room,
and the man we just saw lying on the sidewalk enters the frame (shot 50).
Later in the film she gazes toward the wall in front of her, offscreen (shots
252, 255, and 259), and the death's-head moth appears on the screen (shots
253, 254, 256, 257, 258, and 260), and then the man again (shot 261).

There is a substantial difference between the two gazes, however. The
woman's gaze submits the man's to its dictate, to the point that his gaze be-

comes the product of the woman's in a twofold manner: (a) because the gaze of the man is generated by the woman's gaze physically as device, and (b) because the woman's gaze grants the man's gaze the capability to create a relationship between signifiers whose meaning the man had seemed unable to comprehend. A thorough analysis of the film's development from shot 55 will show that the series of dissolves that break the stupor with which the man stares at the ants crawling on his hand is generated by a play on gazes in which the woman's gaze is the dominant one.

The series begins with both characters looking at the man's hand (shot 55). Immediately after that, a cut shows a close-up of the man's hand (shot 56), whose meaning is as opaque as that of a shot we have just seen (shot 51). In shot 57, the perspective is radically different. The shot begins with the woman looking toward the man's eyes, as he keeps staring at the palm of his hand (shot 57a); the man turns his head and looks at the woman's eyes (shot 57b); the woman turns her eyes toward his hand (shot 57c) and so does the man (shot 57d). When this happens, the hand, shown again in close-up (shot 58), is no longer an object enclosed in its own opacity, for it materially produces through a series of dissolves a swimmer's armpit, a sea urchin, and the sequence of the young woman poking at a severed hand on the street (shots 59, 60, and 61). The third close-up of the hand is not associated through editing with the man's gaze, but with the direction that the woman's gaze imposes on it. This shot acts retrospectively on the relationship between shots 49 and 50 and, in turn, between the one established in shots 252 to 261.

In shots 49 and 50, the woman's gaze summons the man's presence in the room, as a physical materialization of a phantasmic desire explicitly stated in the juxtaposition of shots 45/46 and 47/48. In these shots the disordered pieces of clothing on the bed take the shape of an invisible body, whose weight is made visible by the slight caving-in of the pillow right where the head would be. In shots 252 to 261, and as a correlative of the two examples we have just commented upon (the hand crawling with ants and the woman staring at the bed), the woman's gaze produces an element — the death's-head moth or "skull," as the script states — whose symbolic function is double: it establishes a relationship both with the woman's self-awareness and sexual repression and with her suppression of her relationship with the man. In both cases the story we are watching takes place exclusively in the woman's head, as projection of her desire, or, more concretely, of the analysis the woman makes in the course of the film of her own desire and frustration.[10]

The appearance first of the cyclist in close-up and then of the woman in the bedroom after the intertitle *Eight years later* may seem to question what has just been stated. The causal relationship we pointed out before does not seem to apply. Yet, what we have just mentioned about the man's fictitious physicality as existing only as projection of the woman's gaze will still hold. The temporal inversion in the narrative presentation of the woman's story — the articulation of her ghosts — as flash-forward sends back to marks of the narrator's discourse, not to the structure of the narrated events. Moreover, this inversion can be understood as inscription of the model elaborated in the prologue, that is, as inscription of the metaphor placed in syntagma at the very beginning of the narrative within the narrative comprising the central part of the film. We shall return to this issue at the end of this chapter, when we discuss the false female point of view as male construction.

An Erotic Phantasy; or, How the Dream of Sublimation Produces Monsters

If we take what was stated in the previous section as our hypothesis of departure, we shall notice that the apparent disjointed — or surreal — quality of the story the film seems to narrate has a logic that is at times overwhelming.

The beginning of this story is located, strictly speaking, in shot 22. A woman sitting in the middle of a room stares at a book in which, we find out a little later (shot 26), there is a copy of Vermeer's *The Lacemaker*, a rather evident metaphorical translation of Penelope's myth.[11] Enclosed in her home like Penelope, the woman daydreams, indefinitely postponing — it does not matter at this point whether willingly or not — to act out her desire for a presence of which she becomes aware only at the moment of irremediable loss. It is not by chance that the shots that show the falling of the cyclist are intercut with shots of the woman in the room exactly when the man falls on the sidewalk.

At this moment the woman puts the book aside and confronts the facts. The man is lying motionless on the ground. She (who later will reject all attempts of physical approach) kisses and caresses him passionately over and over again, as one would caress an inanimate object or a puppet incapable of any movement. She picks up the box that was hanging from the cyclist's neck and, in one of the most explicit metaphors of penetration ever shown on screen, puts the key in the lock, uncovering the box's supposed secret. As always happens when a secret is unveiled, there is nothing special in the box.

This is no Pandora's box. With the objects from the box, a necktie and a collar that are different from the ones the cyclist was wearing when he fell, the woman creates her ghost, a ghost capable of taking the place of the real body that fell on the street. The metonymical displacement from the character to his attributes (the striped necktie recalls that of the man with the razor and sends back metaphorically to both the transversal razor edge and the violence associated with it) leaves no doubts about the woman's need to construct her own object. Such operation is carried out, not by chance, on a bed. The man that emerges from nothingness in the middle of the room immediately after this bears none of these attributes — he wears an open shirt and no necktie — and can therefore be objectified with no danger. The hand with the crawling ants produces as a result of the woman's gaze — *not of the man's*, as we have just seen — three successive images equally related to sexuality: an armpit, which is simultaneously a metonymical displacement for the female genitals and also their visual metaphor; a sea urchin, symbol of the seductiveness and destructiveness attributed to physical love by many of the texts of the time, such as, for example, the beginning of Luis Cernuda's *Donde habite el olvido* (Where oblivion dwells; 1934);[12] and a severed hand tossed around with a stick at safe distance by a young woman, who seems to feel attraction and repulsion toward the hand at the same time, another patent metaphorical rendering of the ambivalent feelings of attraction and repulsion accompanying masturbatory practice.

If we emphasize that the original script stated very clearly that the severed hand's fingernails are enameled, even though this detail was not kept in the shooting, it is clear that the hand was meant to be feminine. In spite of the fact that this is not a hypothesis about authorial intention, but a datum from the script, the absence of this detail in the finished product can be explained in meaningful terms from within the textual space of the film.

If we are not surprised that a woman's hand emerges from the woman's gaze, we should remember that this hand may as well be the man's, as it is also looked at by the man (after all, it starts out being his own hand). The ambiguous androgyny of the young woman on the street could therefore be understood as the underscoring of a common trajectory shared by the male and the female from onanism to heterosexuality. In fact, this is what the whole film eventually is about.

The policeman's recriminations (less explicit in the film than in the script) would thus send back to the presence of an order that takes the role of moral watchman and prompts to forsake such sinful habits. From this perspective the policeman is connected, from within the film's textual system, with other marks that recall the image of authority and order: the double (segments 9 to 11) that removes the man's fetishes and represses him in a patent way;[13] the two Marist brothers, who prevent him from approaching the woman; the man in the meadow, and so on.

In their schools, the Marist brothers taught their young students the systematic fear of sex, based on the disastrous and incalculable effect it was supposed to bring upon the health of the soul and the body; one notion they presented with the greatest frequency in their explanations of the diabolical quality of sex was that masturbation caused gangrene and the subsequent detachment of the genitals. Such castration phantasy and its explicit repressive character may perhaps help explain why sexuality is associated to the main characters' impossibility for self-fulfillment. In the night sequence, the sound of the doorbell is suggested by intercutting the images of the man ringing the doorbell with two hands shaking a cocktail mixer (shots 173 and 175), a clear allusion to masturbation. The two shots seem Dalí's suggestion; he later returned to the subject in 1930 with a painting and a literary text, both titled *The Great Masturbator*. Buñuel also would deal with the subject repeatedly. The metaphor is perhaps the most explicit in *Tristana*. In one of the film's final sequences, after her operation, Tristana (Catherine Deneuve) drops her underwear and artificial leg on the bed and leans out of a window, which resembles the niche of a temple, shot as it is in a very low angle shot. She represents the image of the perverse virgin for the desiring eyes of Saturna's son, who is hidden behind the underbrush in the background and stares persistently at the woman's naked body.[14]

The relationship between religion, eroticism, and repression already inscribed in *Un Chien andalou* through the presence of the Marist brothers will be a constant in Buñuel's later films. The question is that if, as Bataille stated, God does not exist, but his corpse is disturbing, then the loss of faith did not bring forth the disappearance of the rhetorical and iconographic universe that the faith implied. Besides underscoring the presence of certain constants and obsessions, this can also be read in another way. In his conversations with Max Aub (1985), Buñuel stated that he did not understand African art or the art of other cultures, and that his reference system had always been the European, Catholic cultural tradition. Thus, compared to the supposed universalism—or ahistoricity—of the vanguardist claims, his work never generalizes; it always deals with specific situations within specific social and cultural systems in order not to affect a folkloric localism that he always despised, but, because of his faithfulness to the postulates of historical materialism, that he never gave up.

The androgyne's death thus comes to represent—like the image of the death's-head moth with which it has a clear syntagmatic relationship—the end of one relationship and the beginning of a new one, even though the man and the woman have two different perspectives in the two instances.

We said earlier that this twofold process of death and rebirth is inscribed in the film's textual system as product of the man's gaze, the only gaze that is shown in countershot as watching from the window while the young woman is knocked down.[15] This does not prevent the male gaze from being shown, in turn, as a projection of the female gaze according to the logic established by the editing; this implies that the events triggered by the androgyne's death are indeed the materialization of the woman's desire.

The result is not exactly what she seems to have hoped for, however, because the man makes the woman the object of an unwonted act of violence. The sequences of the two pianos and of the double that follow the man's decided and virulent attack have the function of articulating some kind of justification for his behavior on the part of the woman. Both sequences are produced, like the previous one, by the woman's desire, a desire that now manifests itself as a will to comprehend and which, therefore, does not resort to ready-made articulations, but generates them in the shape of an argumentation that is not less evident for the fact of having been elided.

Even though they differ in structure and reach, both sequences have a similar function in relation to the shots that present us with the seduction or rape attempt. With regard to the first block (the sequence with the pianos), the man looks down at the floor and picks up two ends of rope in shot 134 as a result of the woman's scornful gaze (shot 132). In the same way we shall see that, if we consequently apply the causal logic that is at work in the film's textual mechanism, the two corkboards from which the pianos, the Marist brothers, and the dead donkeys will successively emerge in perfect *raccord* follow in turn the woman's surprised and appalled look (shot 135). The presence of this series of shots is justified by the necessity to give the bewildered female character an explication: the grand pianos, the Marist brothers, and the dead donkeys may very well be an indirect allusion to the debris of the inherent decadence of bourgeois culture, where art, religion, and putrefaction go hand in hand in articulating a system of values that Buñuel attacked relentlessly and mercilessly; a system of values that most importantly, especially in the present context, is based and thrives on the articulation of sexuality, brutality, and repression. (Thus the ironic reference to Juan Ramón Jiménez's *Platero* in this context—about whose symptomatic value Buñuel and Dalí wrote a most virulent text—exceeds the limits of a merely "vanguardist" provocation.[16])

The series of photograms ends with the image of the hand crawling with ants (shot 163), thus constituting a symmetrical closing for the whole sequence. As a matter of fact, shot 164, where another one of the woman's gazes causes the man to appear once more (shot 165), places the action in the same space that we seem to have just left. Something has changed, however. The man now wears a striped necktie and a collar. He looks the same as before, but now his distinctive traits are those that the woman has imposed on him: he is wearing all the items of clothing that she had previously spread on the bed. In this sense we could say that as a character and in his relationship with the woman, he now represents not only a presence, but also a behavior. Once both scenarios have come together, the woman no longer acts—for the first time in the film—as motor of someone else's action, to whose result she only takes a passive part, but instead is the events' initiator. When the doorbell rings again, she moves across the room to open the door, whereas the man lying in bed is prey of a passivity and bewilderment that prevent him from moving.

After opening the door, the woman disappears from the screen—that is, from the symbolic scenario she has generated—until the end of the sequence, leaving the two men by themselves. Her physical absence does not imply a "real" absence from what we are about to watch; her absence inscribes her presence as the implicit spectator of the events. The connection established in the opening segment between her face and the gaze of the film's spectator is still present in this sequence, and explains the expression of disappointment we see on her face in shot 251, as a result of the ultimate male failure—a failure, let's not forget, whose outcome she could not physically see.

Whether we interpret the newcomer as the "adult double" of the character of the opening sequence or as a stand-in for the father figure, the sequence narrates his failed attempt to get rid of the traumas linked to both possibilities. The two hands shaking the cocktail mixer in shots 173 and 175 can therefore determine a rebellion against what is considered to be the irruption of the "other"—father or adult—as censor of the so-called solitary vice. Hence the transformation of the books into guns (patent and simple metaphor of the instrumental function of learning and culture in the process of growing up, defined by Freud with the graphic expression of "killing the father") allows the literal killing of the image of the repressive "double." It is not by chance that this death triggers two simultaneous false openings: (a) from the inner space, metaphor of the mother's womb, to the outside space (the falling body is then the father image as interiorized by the main character, rather than the father's body); and (b) from the clothed body of the woman (which is undressed only in the man's imagination, when he can look at it, stripped of all garments, with his blinded eyes; shots 112 to 120), to the naked bust of the same woman seated in the meadow. In the latter opening, it is evident that the goal has not been achieved: the woman's body disappears before he can achieve any kind of possession of her. In the case of the former opening, the man appears inside the room again, when the woman's gaze summons him, in shot 261.

The pointlessness of either failed opening is underscored by the explicit lack of interest that the man in the meadow shows for the fallen body. A new representation of power that can be linked metonymically to the father figure, he is the person whom everyone thinks is to be informed of the events, yet he does not even deign to look at how the man's corpse is picked up and carried somewhere else (shots 246b and 246c).

Shot 251 picks up the story line from shot 179. The woman enters the room once more while the sound track underscores her return to the point of departure by accompanying the action not with Wagner's score but with the tango that had been used as background music in the sequence of the attempted seduction/rape.

Up to this point two death scenes have brought about two failed attempts to openings:

(a) the androgyne's death, which led to an attempt to a heterosexual relationship as an alternative to onanism;
(b) the father figure's death, which led to an attempt to a normalized, nontraumatic relationship with the outside world.

In both scenes the woman is a mere passive object of the events. This is when the moth enters the picture. The symbolism is perhaps commonsensical, yet no less poignant because of that. The moth dies to be reborn as a caterpillar: the death it symbolizes therefore refers back to the possibility for a new beginning rather than to an end.[17] The relationship established between this shot and the one showing Vermeer's *Lacemaker* needs no further commentary. The action of spinning and unraveling no longer means an eternal return to the beginning in a neurotically repeated movement; it is now a metaphor for a universe of possible self-transformation.

The woman therefore moves one more step forward *toward her own active opening*. She does not limit herself to the opening of a door in order for someone to come in and decide on her behalf in an enclosed space; rather, she underscores her will to transform by opening the door. She goes out to a space that is clearly a beach—a borderless space and a sexual symbol that seems to have been taken from an introductory manual to Freudianism—where a different man awaits her. In spite of the simplicity of the procedure, it is very clear which interpretive line the film's textual strategy proposes for the text's reading.

We have commented that the image of the moth was to be related structurally to the androgyne's death. In both instances death is related to and identified with birth, and a causal relationship is established between the two. In the case of the moth's image, though, such identification is perceived only by the woman. According to the logic of the shot/countershot previously established, the man is situated in the same space as the moth, with which he could eventually be identified in the eye of the woman: only the man's (symbolic) death or—which amounts to the same—the end of the repressed relationship between the woman and the man's image could create the possibility, already twice aborted, of a real relationship, desired but unfeasible until that moment. What the man does, however, is to erase his mouth—his sexuality—and accept from a distance the image of the woman's genitals (the hair of her armpit) as he looks at her as a voyeur. The tight connection established throughout the film between the notions of voyeurism and repression finds confirmation here in the man's seeing or touching the woman's naked body only when his power of seeing is undercut (shots 114, 117, 236, and 237). Voyeurism and self-fulfillment are shown as incompatible in the film.

In the shots immediately preceding these of the "transplant" of the armpit hair, the woman furiously puts lipstick on her lips as affirmation of her point of view and as a counterpoint to the erasure of the man's mouth at the beginning of the sequence. Just as the sea urchin was a reference to Cernuda's poetics, this sequence seems to make reference to Aleixandre's rhetoric in *Espadas como labios* (1932), where sexual attraction ("labios") is connected to death ("espadas") as the two inseparable sides of the erotic relationship.[18] In front of the man's failures, she can, like a moth, get over the traumas (of life, of sexuality, and so on) and be *other*.

The woman's behavior on the beach is therefore also *other*, yet not different from her behavior with the fallen cyclist. She is the one that approaches, kisses, and caresses this character who, in turn, lets himself be seduced and takes the passive role that the woman had played earlier. The frilly cuffs, skirt, cap, the strap, and the box appear once more on the beach, but now they are dead symbols that refer to nothing and evoke nothing. The new couple can now walk happily toward their spring.

"Woman" Was a Man; or, The *Mise en abyme*

The film develops almost until its end in a seemingly systematic, albeit non-linear, way. Shot 290, the film's last before the closing intertitle, suddenly breaks the logic that had been established until that moment. A freeze frame shows, with an obvious reference to Millet's *Angelus*, the woman and the main male character buried up to their chests in the sand. The man who had walked with the woman along the beach has disappeared.[19]

If we take this image to be the marker of the story's end—which indeed it is—the question is, what kind of story is this? It is clear that the film is not really about the story we have attempted to reconstruct through a rearticulation of the various sequences of the middle block.

If we go back to the film's beginning, to the explicit presence of the director-narrator, we shall be able to reconsider and underscore the fact that if the main male character is the product of the woman's gaze, the woman is in turn the product of the gaze of the man who, behind the camera, observes and articulates the events; that is to say, of the man who constructs through editing the film as a whole. It is not just a woman's point of view; it is, rather, the point of view of a man attempting to capture and articulate, from his own perspective and system of values, what he *believes* to be a woman's point of view.

This rather self-evident reflection has two important consequences. The first is the underscoring of a presence in charge of controlling the order of discourse and therefore of the text's proposals for sense. The second is the imposing on the woman's gaze and on the product of her gaze—*her story*—certain marks that connect her story to the more general and comprehensive story that this man is narrating.

One of Buñuel's own literary texts can perhaps cast light on what we have just mentioned. "Caballería rusticana," included in Sánchez-Vidal (1982), reads as follows:

> In the midst of a truncated afternoon without landscape or a faraway moon, a withered tree twitched its imploring branches, stretching them out toward the inflexible mirror of the sky, repeating endlessly its atrocious gesture.
>
> Over the intact rope of the horizon, three motionless shepherds without consciousness or crook placed an enigmatic vignette to the incredible dusk.
>
> Why don't the two thin afternoon oars—light and shade—furrow the air or design shapes?

Desolation sobbed intermittently as a star breathed its last breath in the remotest corner of the sky.

There was no house, no flight, no stream.

We were three brothers. He, she, and I.

$$HE = SHE$$
$$SHE = I$$
$$HE = I$$

We were three twins. Never did crystal kisses blossom on our foreheads under our roof. It is sad and humiliating to speak of it, we were three parthenogenetic twins.

This is what happened one afternoon, or rather *that* truncated afternoon without landscape or a faraway moon.

Leaning against the Gothic window—the dwelling's only source of light—she had waved him good-bye for a while with the white caress of her little kerchief, until she saw him disappear in the distance. Then she sat by the fire where she would spin, diluting the hours with her gazes; the murmuring of the streams kept her company, and she remained a virgin, as required by her maidenhood.

Yet the ominous foreboding of the afternoon weighed down her heart with the monotonous and inflexible swinging of a pendulum.

Suddenly the garden barked. Someone was walking along the street.

Ah! . . . At last.

HE came back. It was about six. But he came back without HER. Where did he leave her? What had he done with her chaste cheerfulness? In what gloomy minute did SHE merge forever with the mysterious, frightening afternoon, as forlorn and irremediable as the past?

Terrified, holding my breath, I did not dare ask when I saw her come in. The day's death rattle still trembled in her eyes.

My brother dropped his old Arabic rifle in a corner and began sobbing by the fire.

My god, what anguish!

"How could you, brother, to HER, our sister . . . "

He writhed in pain without a cry. Tears rolled copiously down his face; they thickened by his cheeks and on his chest before falling on the ground. They were burning tears, tears of wax, and his regret was as intense as a flame quivering over his head. All of him was melting as a candle now.

Tied up, elbow to elbow, darkness entered the dwelling.

A first reading of the text reveals the occurrence of certain elements and images also present in the film: the image of the young woman spinning by the window as in Vermeer's *Lacemaker*,[20] the sudden awareness that someone is coming in from the outside to break the inflexible monotony of the passing of time, the discovery that such presence from the outside world will not make any difference whatsoever, and so on. But besides these superficial similarities with the film's subject matter, a reading of this text also allows something else: the nonidentification between the characters and the "I" that unifies and speaks them.

In the literary text an "I" is waiting for a woman. However, when the man (HE) arrives, SHE has disappeared and the narrating "I" has taken her place. We therefore have the objectified splitting of the narrative's only omniscient voice, the voice of the "I." Another element relevant to our purpose is the definition of the female character as innocent victim—"How could you, brother, to HER, our sister . . . " The procedure is the same as that used later in *Un Chien andalou*, even though the explicitness of the written word may seem to come through in what has been read as the film's classical narrative structure.

Woman is connected to a certain negativity in her relationship with man in Buñuel's oeuvre; this comes through rather clearly in his later films, such as *Susana, Subida al cielo, Viridiana*, and *Tristana*. Such negativity, however, does not derive from the woman's (supposed) utter culpability; it is, rather, the outcome of her total innocence, or—what amounts to the same—of her radical, and positively subversive, amorality.[21] At the same time, she is called to play the part of the victim within the role division imposed by society. Only when she rids herself of patriarchal morality—it does not matter whether this morality is imposed by men or women, because it is interiorized as one's own—can she look at the world with new eyes, from her own point of view. Thus Susana is less the negative character that is to be sent back to jail, than the triggerer of a crisis in those values that her presence shows to be hypocritical and deceitfully stable. Tristana plays the role of executioner only as a reaction to those structures that curtail her freedom. Either when these women are fully aware and in control of their situations, or when they feel compelled to submit themselves to the circumstances, as in the case of Viridiana, their desires to be free necessarily imply the questioning of the system of values of Western culture, the only value system to which Buñuel refers explicitly and among whose norms he sets his characters—away, as we remarked before, from abstract or metaphysical generalizations.

Another text by Buñuel, belonging to the same period as "Caballería rusticana," summarizes very well the point I am attempting to make.

A Decent Story

Carmencita was very docile. Her innocence was proverbial. Her mother watched over her night and day, raising in front of her daughter the wall of her vigilance against the lures of the world. When Carmencita turned twelve, her mother became very concerned. "The day my daughter menstruates *for the first time*," she thought, "that'll be the end of her golden innocence." But she managed to resolve the problem. When she saw Carmencita turn pale for the first time, she went out to the street like a madwoman and came back a little later with a big bunch of red flowers. "Take this, darling, you are becoming a woman." And Carmencita, deceived and happy with those wonderful red flowers, forgot to menstruate. Every month, twelve times a year and for many years, Carmencita was deceived and preserved from the terrible truth. Whenever those black circles around her eyes seemed to forerun the end of each month, her mother gave her red flowers.

Carmencita turned forty. Her mother, who was now very old, still called her Carmencita, even though everybody else called her Lady Carmela. When she was that age, the month arrived when Carmencita had no black circles around her eyes, and her mother gave her a bouquet of white flowers. "Take this, darling, this is the last bunch I shall give you, for now you are no longer a woman." "But mother, I never even realized that I was one," Carmencita objected. Her mother replied: "So much the worse for you, darling." That white bouquet, rotten, leafless, scattered, and withered, was what they placed in Carmencita's coffin.[22]

An Indecent Story

When Mariquita was close to the critical age, her mother wanted to do the same as with Carmencita, and when she saw black circles around her eyes and saw her turn pale, she gave her a bunch of red roses. But Mariquita was much bolder than Carmencita. She grabbed the flowers, opened the window, flung them out, and menstruated.[23]

Un Chien andalou presents us with a similar setting. Buñuel himself slits the woman's eye, therefore forcing her to see with different eyes. This may indeed constitute the prologue's fifth function: to force the gaze to make its own narrative, to produce its own liberation, something quite different from the militant reductionism with which Jean-Louis Perrier (1969) connected the slitting of the eye with "a univocal, petit bourgeois rasping operation, an anarchist temptation to resolve all contradictions from the outside, pointing to Breton's ideal place from where all contradictions cease to be perceived as such."

If we return to the prologue and to the inversion Linda Williams pointed out, which is produced from within the metaphorical structure of shots 1 to 4 and 8 to 12, we shall notice how such inversion can be traced in the whole film. As we remarked earlier, shots 13 to 21 precede the first inscription of the woman's look. If the male character is the "seen object," we have here the relationship "object + gaze" that characterized shots 1 to 4. In shots 22 to 289—that is, all of the story within the story, and up to shot 289—the relationship is "gaze + object." This is what we had in shots 8 to 12, the shots that showed us the slitting of the eye; at this moment the woman can finally see things as they are, apart from the function assigned to them by patriarchal tradition and by the system of values that this tradition underpins. The rhyme effect these shots create with shots 114 and 116 is therefore neither gratuitous nor fortuitous.

In short, the narrator's explicit determination indicates how to read the film by inverting the "metaphor placed insyntagm," to use Linda Williams's appropriate expression, and at the same time provides the keys to understanding his ineludible presence in the prologue itself, from the film's very beginning, which thus foretells not only the film's future development at the level of the story line, but also its structure and textual mechanism.

The film's third and last part closes the circle by referring back to the prologue as totality. It is not by chance, therefore, that this part consists of one freeze frame. In the prologue the narrator imposed the opening necessary for the woman's story to be produced by the woman herself; now his own gaze, frozen as image, closes and closures such story by bringing the stream of sense to the narrative's origin. The happy ending marking the liberation of the two characters on the beach as the epitome of the heterosexual couple (produced by the woman's point of view) gives way to a less "happy" ending (from the narrator's point of view), or at least to a more ambiguous one (the woman keeps on looking up, the man looks down), which neutralizes the happy ending and/or makes both endings equivalent.

Fragmentation; or, Talking about Love

In the article "*Découpage* o segmentación cinegráfica" (Sánchez-Vidal, 1982), Buñuel advances some considerations that may be useful to emphasize now. After declaring the nonexistence of the "actor" (in a strict sense of the word) in cinema,[24] he writes:

The film's intuition, the photogenic embryo, throbs already in the process we call découpage. Segmentation. Creation. Something splits to become something else. What did not exist before, exists now. An act—the most simple and the most complicated one—of procreation, of creation. From the ameoba to a symphony. It is the film's truest moment of creation, creation through fragmentation. In order for this process to be enacted in cinema, it will require a segmentation in fifty, a hundred-odd pieces. They will follow one another vermicularly and, by arranging themselves in colonies, will constitute the film's body, a big tapeworm of silence made of material segments (the editing) and of the ideal one (découpage). Segmentation of segmentation . . . An isolated image represents very little. A simple, unstructured monad, where evolution stops and continues at the same time. A direct transcription of the world: a filmic larva . . . The lens—this amoral, unprejudiced eye without tradition, capable nevertheless to interpret by itself—sees the world. The filmmaker orders it later. Machine and human being . . . A good film with good photography and excellent camera work and cast but without a good découpage would result, as a whole, into something nonphotogenic, as a good collection of animated photos. As the sounds produced by a big orchestra before the performance are incommensurably different from the symphony itself, as distant is such ensemble of images from resembling a film. But the opposite can happen: a film without characters but with natural objects, with a mediocre photography, may be a good film . . . The filmmaker . . . is such not so much at the moment of the shooting as in the supreme moment of segmentation.

I would like to underscore three basic ideas present in this text that articulate not only the technical aspects of the weltanschauung expressed in *Un Chien andalou*, but also, fundamentally, the compositional methodology that structured it. First, there is the relationship established between segmenting (to cut, to break a unity) with reproduction and (re)birth; second, the explicit subjection of the thematic elements to the idea of structure, that is, to the "order of discourse"; and third, the attendant dissolution of the camera eye's neutrality—as amoral, unprejudiced eye—which is integrated and subsumed to the filmmaker's point of view.

We have already discussed the discursive functioning of such notions. Now I would like to deal with the analysis of the way in which, coherently with the foundational principle that unifies them (form does not have a ground, it produces it), such principles produce the story narrated in the film.

If we accept the thesis Dénis de Rougemont elaborates in his well-known book *L'amour et l'Occident* (*Love in the Western World*), the general idea that has dominated literature in particular and, in general, Western culture as a whole is that love involves the transgression of the law. The renowned medieval poem *Tristan and Isolde* would lead this hypothesis to the extreme: all love is adulterous. It is therefore quite significant that Buñuel chose for the film's sound track precisely the score by Wagner that is based on the medieval love story, and that he complemented it with tango music, so much related to stories about adultery, desertion, and unfaithfulness.[25]

In this way, the breaking of the law is the condition sine qua non of the love relationship. The shadow cast by the presence of a third party (husband, wife, the law) and the attendant threat of punishment make such relationship, sheltered by secret, a source of unsuspected pleasure. This pleasure has everything to do with loss of identity, with the dissolution of the social "I" into the pure materiality of the bodily and individualized "I."

William Shakespeare expressed it, with the mastery characteristic of all his works, in what is perhaps his best elaboration of the topic, *Romeo and Juliet*, as Julia Kristeva (1987) pointed out in a thought-provoking essay. When Juliet discovers that the man she is in love with belongs to an enemy family, her words are most explicit:

> 'Tis but thy name that is my enemy;
> Thou art thyself, though not a Montague.
> What's Montague? It is nor hand, nor foot,
> Nor arm, nor face, nor any other part
> Belonging to a man . . .
>   doff thy name;
> And for thy name, which is no part of thee,
> Take all myself.
>
> (2.2.38–49)

The characters in *Un Chien andalou* do not have to give up their names, because they do not even have any. In the space left vacant by the first linking with the social "I," the process of liberation will take place, that is, the access to a pleasure that the female character seems to be longing for without being able to attain.[26]

To give up one's name is in this case a metaphor for the loss of one's own identity, that is, the loss of the social unity called "I." This is why it is associated both with fragmentation—the quartering of one's self and of the other—and with the substitution of the metaphor of the day (the space of the law) by the metaphor of the night (the space where the law can be erased or transgressed), with the substitution of the metaphor of the sun by the metaphor of the moon.

if love be blind,
It best agrees with night. Come, civil night . . .
Give me my Romeo; and, when he shall die,
Take him and cut him out in little stars . . .

(3.2.9–22)

We have already commented on the relationship established in *Un Chien andalou* between erotic fulfillment and the undercutting of the power of the gaze. Fragmentation now seems an even more important issue. In the text mentioned at the beginning of this section Buñuel defined the film's découpage as the procedure by means of which something is split so that it can become something else. Not only will this principle affect the film's structural mechanism, it will also justify the apparent gratuitousness of some of the shots: the woman recomposes the man's image with parts that define him metaphorically—the frilly cuffs, cap, and skirt, the collar, the necktie, the box; her desire to turn onanism into a heterosexual relationship produces the symbolic cutting off and hurling of the man's hand. All of her story is likewise generated through the articulation of scattered fragments freely combined together by the logic of her desire. From this perspective the story we are told can be read as an initiating journey from the familial order (whose symbol is the room) to the space of an uncoded relationship that does not repress and is determined by choice (the beach, a new man, and so on).

It is rather interesting to note how Buñuel analyzes his characters' repressions and frustrations by placing them in enclosed spaces. This will be the norm in all his later films and is a procedure that is not fortuitous but premeditated, as the filmmaker himself admitted to Max Aub (1985). Such enclosed spaces, whether physical (*The Exterminating Angel, The Discreet Charm of the Bourgeoisie*) or mental (*This Strange Passion, Simon of the Desert*), seem to point to a conception of the world—the world as a discursive, historically analyzable construct—as a prison that no one and nothing can ultimately escape. This is why the "adjustment" implied by the passage from the onanistic relationship to the adult order of heterosexuality is also not a solution; such relationship is part of this prison-world and is also submitted to its rules, as the final shot of *Un Chien andalou* most explicitly states. Mutilation, one of the topics present in all of Buñuel's later films and whose metaphorical climax occurs with Tristana's severed leg, is therefore only a form of fragmentation, understood as the only path to the love relationship.

The connection established by juxtaposing day and night in the opening

segment and the sequence of the "double" is significant. In the opening segment, the slitting of the eye is directly connected to a space at night,
metaphorically represented by the full moon; in the sequence of the "double," the action takes place "about 3 A.M." In both situations the transgression carried out at night gives way to a "new" day: the woman can now see
how to get out of her impasse. The soft gray hue of the final freeze frame that
follows in a contradictory way the sign "in spring," would refer back, according to this reading, to the ambivalence that the narrator sees in this possibility. The narration of the transformational process is, from his perspective, the history of a discovery that is as necessary as it is useless.

Ado Kyrou (1963) remarked that a constant feature in Buñuel's filmic
texts is the structuring of three different stages: an opening sequence structured as a prologue, where the rules of the game are laid down; a middle part,
where the story develops in a more or less complete way; and an epilogue,
usually brief and unexpected, which surprises the viewer by questioning the
logical ending or by inverting it, as if the director refused to closure his films
with clear-cut denouements or conclusions.

Thus the abrupt ending of *Land without Bread*, with the main character's
corpse falling in a dung heap, recalls conceptually the hurried ending of *La
mort dans ce jardin* or the explosion at the end of *That Obscure Object of
Desire*, to mention two extreme and quite different examples.

Un Chien andalou foreruns such strategy with shot 290. Buñuel's tragic
skepticism, so evident in all of his later works, is already prefigured in this
short film, which seems to state, as Cioran would write in later years, that
the main feature of the love relationship is that it makes no difference between happiness and unhappiness.

Chapter Three
A Writing of Disorder:
The Discursive Proposal of
Un Chien andalou

> *It was necessary for our dear eyes, our dear eyes, to reflect what was not and yet was as intense as the things which actually "are." We needed real images in order to stop missing what we had left behind.*
>
> André Breton, *Le surréalisme et la peinture*

> *Not that cinema must be devoid of all human psychology, on the contrary; but it should give this psychology a far more live and active form, free from the connections which try to make our motives appear idiotic instead of flaunting them in their original and profound barbarity.*
>
> Antonin Artaud

In recent years several books and articles have focused on the well-known polemic between Antonin Artaud and Germaine Dulac about *The Seashell and the Clergyman*.[1] A discussion of this film—considered by Artaud as avatar of Buñuel's *Un Chien andalou* and *The Age of Gold*—and of its relationship with Buñuel's first two films will enable us to tackle the delicate issue of the relationship between surrealism and cinema. A detailed analysis of the cinematic materiality of these films will allow us to resolve the question about whether surrealist cinema did actually exist. In the case of a negative answer—the position I personally endorse—the analysis itself will clarify and explain the reasons for surrealism's nonexistence.

We are faced, then, with the most general problem of the so-called historic avant-gardes, within whose theoretical and referential framework these films have been studied and classified. Octavio Paz (1964) described surrealism as the last great spiritual revolution of the West. Yet, in the late 1960s, one of the most qualified texts of the French situationist movement testifies to surrealism's failure in the following terms: "Dada attempted to destroy art before creating it; surrealism attempted to create it without destroying it."

In his book *Poets, Prophets and Revolutionaries: The Literary Avant-Garde from Rimbaud through Postmodernism*, Charles Russell (1985) pointed out that the origin of the so-called historic avant-gardes—and, in more general terms, of literature and modern art as well—was based on the artist's acknowledgment of the highly problematic and contradictory relationship between the artist's own function and modern society. Artists were at the time immersed into a specific value system that thoroughly determined their work, while they were aware of the antagonistic position of such values vis-à-vis aesthetic experience. According to Russell's study, since the age of romanticism in France, in the last third of the nineteenth century in England, and in most European and American countries at the beginning of the present century, writers and artists were faced with three different alternatives regarding the social role of art and literature. The artist could: (1) be an acritical voice of the dominant value system; (2) articulate an ethical, aesthetic, or spiritual vision at odds with those values, but with the determination to recover or add a meaningful dimension to the existing culture; or (3) attempt to imagine or implement through his or her work a radical change in this society, to which the artists belonged. The first alternative resulted in kitsch forms and popular culture; the second was the propeller of the best of "high culture," that is, of modernism (Joyce, Proust, Mann, Rilke, Musil, Yeats, Stevens, Faulkner, and so on); the third was the basis for the avant-garde movements and the different and specifically political art proposals (Brecht, socialist realism in Russia after the October Revolution, and so on).

The distinction made by Russell between modernist and vanguardist proposals was meant to make distinctions among what had been generally considered as complementary manifestations within one single tradition, subsequent to romanticism, known with the generic term of avant-garde (Poggioli, 1968; Noszlopy, 1969; Paz, 1971). In Russell's view, their differences are due to their different notions of the social function of art:

> It need be stressed that when hermeticism and sociopolitical activism move beyond the mere recognition of a problem and the initial turn toward the creative act, the artists' expectations of the effects of their commitment differ qualitatively. It is here, in the writer's or artist's attitude toward art, the artwork, the creative act itself, and toward the audience and society, that significant psychological differences are evident between writers and artists in the avant-garde and modernist camps. (15)

In effect, while modernism dealt with the issue of social antagonism by integrating it into the artwork as a mere anecdote, the avant-garde, closer to the positions of nihilism, aimed to participate actively in the process of social change. Thus the innovative principles typical of modernists turned into open experimentalism in the avant-garde, and the longing for a transcendental dimension in art and society became an invocation of the visionary powers of the artist. From an epistemological point of view, however, both the modernists and the avant-garde shared a faith in the power of language to affect life and social structures, either through the effects produced on the perception, knowledge, and behavior of each reader or community of readers, or through their cooperation (from their specificity) with other social groups. From a pragmatic point of view, both movements coincided in the belief in art's specificity, that is, in the power of art as such, as a specific field of knowledge. Both accepted the idea of artistic autonomy, and considered this as a base from which to conceive of the artist's social role.

The dogmatic postulates of the Communist leaders in the Soviet Union after 1924 posed numerous problems to the Russian futurists. From the perspective of the Western countries, such problems established a false opposition between free and state art. A country that had achieved a revolution was supposed to be unable to appreciate and understand the literary and artistic achievements of avant-garde, so Western artists and writers were determined to stake their territory in the face of all sorts of impositions, including those perpetrated in the name of Marx, as in the case of Louis Aragon's reaction to criticism by French Communists. History has proved that socialist realism was not able to understand the problems posed by art and literature, at least as far as its results were concerned (altogether not too different from the effects of the ideology of nineteenth-century bourgeois naturalism). Nevertheless, some writers and artists, such as Bertolt Brecht, did offer a different alternative without directly committing themselves to the ideas defended and claimed by the avant-garde. For Brecht, what was at stake in the debate about revolutionary practices in art and literature was not the existence or nonexistence of artistic freedom, but the questioning of the very notion of art. Such questioning implied an analysis of the social conditions that made possible the bourgeois concept of art as we know it.

Surrealism's failure to integrate vanguardism with political practice both at its first (*La Révolution surréaliste*) and second (*Le Surréalisme au service de la Révolution*) stages can be explained as the logical result of its own theoretical presuppositions rather than by the difficult coexistence of art and politics. In any case, the fact that this problematic was confronted one way or another makes surrealism a suitable example for the discussion of this complex issue.

Surrealism has always been linked to two ambiguous and misleading concepts: revolution and avant-garde. The group's leaders considered revolution as a means for extending individual and collective behaviors by breaking the barriers between the conscious and the unconscious, the rational and the irrational, between imagination and reason. It was not a proposal for the actual creation of a new world but *an idea of a new world*. The articulation and implementation of such an idea was a different matter. Fredric Jameson (1981) has pointed out that automatic writing could be understood, at most, as surrealism's model-idea for a reader informed by surrealist notions, who could reach into his or her subconscious by imitating its procedures.

Breton said that Marx's dictum ("Change the world") and Rimbaud's words ("Transform life") meant the same thing to the surrealists. Their practice, however, underscored the contradiction between the different weltanschauungen grounding each statement. For Marx, the problems posed by the historical discourse did not stem from the attempt to define who or what its subject was, but from the analysis of what constituted its "motor." The dehumanization that was implied also meant the dissolution of a central subject as originator of the discourse. For Breton and Philippe Soupault, who were the core of what was to become the surrealist movement, the suspension of self-control and critical reflection in the "creative" act did not imply dehumanization, but something like Rimbaud's "Je est autre," "another" understood as the other side of the personal self, which could be reached once the repressive dominations of reason and of consciousness were eliminated.

It is not surprising that surrealist poetics focused on the lyrical poem, traditionally more suitable to let the "I" express itself without having to be submitted to external formalities supposedly at the origin of the narrative mode. Breton and his group rejected the nineteenth-century novel because its realism only accounted for the discontinuity of consciousness, without integrating the continuity between conscious and unconscious life. In his book *La realidad como sospecha*, Juan-Miguel Company's (1986) analysis of Émile Zola's work proves that this superficial approach is misleading. The fact that the films by Buñuel more directly connected to this issue (*Nazarín* and *Tristana*) are based on two novels by Galdós, seems to support Company's hypothesis.

In spite of surrealists' later claims on Buñuel's films, cinema was not considered a proper medium for their ideas. Its submission to the imperatives of technological rationality and the collective production process imposed by its industrial matrix were, to a certain extent, incompatible with the surrealists' postulates. Which individual and repressed self was supposed to speak in a film?

In 1925, however, Jean Goudal had seen in film a perfectly suitable space for the implementation of the surrealists' project. In his article "Surréalisme et cinéma," Goudal pointed to the main problems in carrying out Breton's ideas about literature and painting: (1) How can we have access to the unconscious without the help of consciousness, if there is an unsurmountable gap between dreams and reality? (2) How can the proposals of antilogicism be put into practice without giving up communication?

Cinema was for Goudal a way out of that impasse. In his article he stated that cinema was able to overcome the first problem thanks to its capability to produce a "conscious hallucination," a state that allowed the fusion between dreams and reality pursued by the surrealists. According to Goudal, when we sit in a movie theater our gaze is captured by the image projected on the screen. Life outside the cinema walls stands still, our daily problems are suspended, our neighbors cease to exist, and we experience a temporary disembodiment. We are just two eyes fixed on a white surface. In this way, cinema is capable of reproducing some of the elements proper to dreams, without obliterating completely the consciousness of the spectator. Something in its mechanisms allows both the awareness that what we see is unreal and the belief in the reality of that illusion.

Goudal declared that the second problem is solved by cinema's ability to produce, through the succession of images, a meaning that has nothing to do with the logic of verbal language. It is important to note here that "avant-garde" is not the same as "elite," even though most movements known as avant-garde were actually more of an "elite" than "avant-garde." To work against the norms of verisimilitude is a hard task carried out by very few people, but this does not mean that its function and effects are limited to those few. The rebellion against nineteenth-century bourgeois art, which may well be considered part of the heritage of avant-garde movements, was not something new or original. Its first manifestations date back to romanticism. At that time, the fight against machines and the dehumanization of relationships (without taking into account Lamartine's or Zorrilla's decadent romanticism, mention should be made of Shelley, Byron, Blake, Hugo, Espronceda) took a very critical turn on two parallel and simultaneous fronts: against *material* and *mental* exploitation. Although progress on the first front was remarkable (*The Communist Manifesto*, organization of mass movements, the Paris Commune, and so on), it did not lead to an equal development of the second front. The success of individualism as an alternative to automatization was eventually integrated as part of the system it was supposed to fight; it was not only encouraged, but also produced by the system in order to create a safety valve to ensure its survival. Nothing is more controllable, in effect, than a kind of marginalization endowed with the marks of the exceptional. When generalized, marginality is a form of subversion; when confined to the individual and automatized, it is only a form of isolation. Also, its sacralization/mythification greatly annuls its power and significance. Emilio Garroni (1974) saw this very clearly: between Duchamp and a nineteenth-century decadent individual, there is an inversion, not a breach. Both tend to "épater les bourgeois," while needing the world they attack in order to exist.

Dadaism reproduced a similar practice in an inverted way, without achieving the only consequent and significant goal: to undo the idea of the mirror and, with that, the notion of bourgeois art as an immediate and necessary reference to understand the specificity of its own endeavor. The assimilable nature of dadaism was what ultimately determined the end of the movement. The gradual co-optation of most of its outstanding members into the artist's traditional status (as the codirector of *Révue Européenne*, Soupault had worked with "orthodox" figures such as Valéry Larbaud and Edmond Jaloux), together with its increasing credibility, led dadaism to the edge of the "literary consecration" (Breton). Yet, dadaists became the victims of their own pitfalls. Despite these factors, the position defended by dada demanded a process of destruction—destruction of composition rules, of the false dichotomy between aesthetic/nonaesthetic materials, of the opposition between art and life—as the artist's most immediate and inevitable task.

The objective of surrealism seems to be the overcoming of this impasse. One subscribes to this thesis when speaking of surrealism as dada's continuation or legitimate descendant. However, the links between the two movements are to be found in dada's transgressive, rather than subversive, nature: the exchange value their marginal condition granted them. A brief quotation from the best-known "fool" of surrealism, Dalí, illustrates this aspect quite effectively: "In these circumstances, Salvador Dalí, with the precise apparatus of paranoic-critical activity in his hand, is most reluctant to abandon his uncompromising cultural stand, and has proposed for some time that surrealities be eaten, since we, the surrealists, are high quality, decadent, stimulating, extravagant, and ambivalent food. This kind of food is the most suitable to the *faisandé*, paradoxical, and exquisitely horrifying condition proper to the ideological and moral confusion we have the honor and pleasure to live in" (Dalí, 1935).

When Dalí published his article, the Bretonian movement was nearly finished (if we assume that, as avant-garde, the experience will have been exhausted with the beginning of World War II). By that time numerous changes and variants had been introduced to the theses of the first manifesto of 1924. However, the quasi-religious character of the group, with its dogmas, excommunications, even a pope, and all this implied for the creation of a privileged elite, was already at the basis of Breton's first text.

Georges Ribemont-Dessaignes wrote in *Déjà-jadis*: "Surrealism was created from one of dada's ribs." When Breton published *Manifesto of Surrealism* in 1924, however, the idea of a strict discipline to channel the artist's work, beyond all liberalism, had already taken the place of the dadaist anarchy, and introduced the notions of order, hierarchy, and power. Dadaism was totally dismantled, nothing of its projects or aspirations still existing. Breton did not deny the value of literature; rather, he proposed the literary exploitation of an unexplored territory: the world of dreams. To that end, so ambiguous a technique called "automatic writing"—a sort of systematization of Tristan Tzara's "dadaist spontaneity"—had to be used. I would like to point out two things in this respect: the first about the antirealism, antinaturalism of the Bretonian project, and the second about its supposed political function, exemplified by the surrealist manifesto of 1924, "above all and always revolution."

We should remember that Nietzsche had already stated that logic as the one and only ruler leads to falsehood, because logic is not the one and only ruler. But there are hardly any links between Nietzsche's systematic subversion and the Bretonian project. The surrealists' goal was not to undermine the Cartesian foundations of Western aesthetic discourse, to which they juxtaposed another competing aesthetic discourse. They did not reject the notion of system; they wanted to constitute another one, thus reinforcing the paradigms imposed by the language of reason, which they needed as an ever-present ghost, as a reference point in order to oppositionally define and make sense of their own practice. So-called automatism was an attempt to break with rational language and everything it implied: the dictates of the norms that are always someone's norms imposing meanings and patterns of behavior. Breton's definition is as follows: "[Surrealism is] psychic automatism in its pure state, by which one proposes to express—verbally, by means of the written word, or in any other manner—the actual functioning of thought. [It is] dictated by thought, in the absence of any control exercised by reason, exempt from any aesthetic or moral concern" (Breton, 1969, 26). Hence the importance granted imagination, although imagination, whether conscious or unconscious, is always considered as a form of memory after all. To think that by running away from reason we run away from the law means to assume that the law has no access to the unconscious; this implies that we can avoid fighting another enemy whose existence is not even recognized as such (this is a mistake Nietzsche did not make). In his often-quoted letter to André Rolland, Breton writes: "We have never supposed any surrealist text to be the perfect example of verbal automatism. Even in the best 'uncontrolled' texts, one can detect some resistances. A minimum control always remains, generally speaking, like a sort of poetic balance."

The "poetic balance" is but the manifest internalization of a norm, one produced historically within a specific tradition whose dominion Breton pretends to escape. To think in terms of an ahistorical norm would lead us to a metaphysical sphere that could hardly be associated to the explicit Marxism informing the view of the group's major theoretician. Breton admits the limits of the surrealist approach, but because he does not recognize them as limits and limitations at the same time, they are never subverted as such. In this sense, the surrealists' support of the October Revolution is not epistemological in nature; it is granted through the marginalized figure of a dissident, Leon Trotsky, whom the surrealists explicitly idealize as a leader. Apart from the fact that he could be considered by the surrealists as the real embodiment of the revolution against Stalin's barbarism, it is obvious that Trotsky's most appealing trait was that he was a dissident: what mattered to the surrealists was the exchange value of his marginalization.

From a literary and artistic point of view, the only productive writing is that which used the Bretonian technique from without, so to speak, that is, with the awareness that its workings and possible accomplishments can serve the purpose of deconstructing its own normative matrix. Surrealists do not add much to a language that is indeed "liberated" more by writers such as e. e. cummings, James Joyce, and William Carlos Williams than by Breton. Indeed, *Nadja* provides a good example of academic prose in the truest tradition of the West.

I believe it was precisely the conscious use of automatism, that is, the possibility to use as a tool what was basically nothing but a composition technique, that made possible the existence of the so-called Spanish surrealism. Luis Cernuda said something to this effect when discussing Vicente Aleixandre on one occasion, but this notion could be understood to be generally true. Surrealism enabled artists to say or do things that otherwise they would not have said or done because of political or moral censorship. At the same time, it widened and made more flexible the institutionalized channels through which the discourse of art could express itself.

A different point of view should be taken with Antonin Artaud's *The Seashell and the Clergyman* and Buñuel's first film. In these cases, the question was not how to express by means of an imagery capable of escaping dominant ideology what that very ideology was capable of subsuming or integrating, but to challenge, question, and disrupt that ideology from within. Here is where we find the concordances and divergences between Artaud and Dulac, between Dulac's film and Buñuel's work, and between Artaud, Dulac, Buñuel, and Breton. Let us examine these issues in detail.

Our first issue has to do with the relationship between Artaud's script of *The Seashell and the Clergyman* and the film as it was shot and edited by Germaine Dulac. The story of the relationship and problems between the director and the scriptwriter is confused and controversial. Initially, it seems that Artaud meant to direct the film himself, but because of the difficulties he encountered in financing the film, he accepted that the film would be directed by Dulac. He praised her in his article "Le cinéma et l'abstraction" (*Le Monde Illustré*, October 1927), which was the official presentation of the project. However, he was not allowed to take any part whatsoever in the preparatory work for the shooting, in the selection of the cast, or in the actual shooting. This resulted in Artaud's deep disagreement with the finished work. He felt that his ideas and the overall meaning of the project had been betrayed. Many critics have underestimated the surrealists' boycott of the premiere of the film at the "Studio des Ursulines" in February 1928, alleging that Artaud never asked to have his name taken away from the credits. His later claims about his own work being the source of Buñuel's first two films and Jean Cocteau's *Le sang d'un poète* were likewise used to turn the disagreements between Artaud and Dulac into an almost personal controversy. I believe, however, that rather than constituting superficial discrepancies, the differences between Artaud's script and Dulac's film stem from two radically different notions of cinema.

It seems clear that Antonin Artaud conceived of the new medium as an apparatus capable of subverting the institutionalized functioning of traditional art:

> The superiority and the power of this art are due to the fact that its rhythm, its speed, its withdrawal from life, its illusory aspect require close sifting and the distillation of the essential nature of all its elements . . .
> The cinema is an amazing stimulant. It acts directly on the gray matter of the brain . . . In the cinema the actor is merely a live symbol. He alone is the stage, the author's idea, and the sequence of events. That is why we do not think about him. Chaplin acts Chaplin, Pickford acts Pickford. Fairbanks acts Fairbanks. They are the film. It would be inconceivable without them. They are in the foreground where they do not get in anybody's way.

That is why they do not exist. So nothing interposes itself any longer between the work and the spectator. ("Reply to an Inquiry," in Artaud, 1972, 3:59–60).

In the cinema I have always distinguished a quality peculiar to the secret movement and matter of images. The cinema has an unexpected and mysterious side which we find in no other form of art . . . Raw cinema, taken as it is, in the abstract, exudes a little of this trance-like atmosphere, eminently favorable for certain revelations. *To use it to tell a story is to neglect one of its best resources, to fail to fulfill its most profound purpose.* ("Witchcraft and the Cinema" in Artaud, 1972; 3:65–66; emphasis added)

In his letters, twelve texts, and seven scripts, Artaud proposes a new and subversive concept of cinema, one that clearly differs from the dominant modes of representation of the time.[2] His becoming uninterested in cinema at the beginning of the 1930s has not allowed the proper acknowledgment of his importance for film history. The extraordinary success of *Un Chien andalou* and *The Age of Gold* on the one hand and, on the other, the ambiguous relationship between his script for *The Seashell and the Clergyman* and the film as it was directed and edited by Germaine Dulac have also not helped to do justice to this remarkable figure.

If we were to define succinctly the difference between the two stages of the filmmaking process (script and finished film), we could resort to the distinction made by Artaud himself between vanguardism of form (film) and vanguardism of content (script). At a first viewing, the film of *The Seashell and the Clergyman* seems to follow quite (or maybe too) faithfully Artaud's script. The question, though, is not the director's faithfulness in her translation of Artaud's words into images, but rather the problem posed by conceiving the problem in terms of translation, and the film's own subjection to certain individual elements, detrimental to the overall structure of the film as work in progress. Two examples can help clarify this point: the film's opening sequence and the sequence of the confessional booth.

Artaud describes the opening sequence as follows:

The lens discloses a man dressed in black, busy pouring a liquid into glasses of various sizes and volumes. He does this with a sort of oyster shell and breaks the glasses after having used them. The accumulation of flasks next to him is incredible. At one point a door opens and there appears a debonaire-looking officer, complacent, bloated and overloaded with medals. He drags an enormous sabre behind him. He appears like a sort of spider, now in dark corners, now on the ceiling. With each new broken flask the officer makes another hop. But now the officer is behind the man dressed in black. He takes the oyster shell from his hands. The man looks on in peculiar astonishment. The officer goes around the room a few times with the shell, then, suddenly drawing his sword from its scabbard, he shatters the shell with a gigantic blow. The whole room trembles. The lamps flicker and in each trembling reflection gleams a sabre point. The officer walks out heavily and the man dressed in black, who looks very like a clergyman, goes out after him on all fours. (*The Shell and the Clergyman*, in Artaud, 1972, 3:21–22)

In the film, after the credits[3] and before the close-up of the shoulder of a man dressed in black, a long shot shows a half-open door through which the light reaches a dark hall. Thus, from the very beginning, there is a clear intention to narrativize the sequence by diegetizing the camera's point of view. There is, therefore, a transition from the script's *objective camera* to the film's *subjective camera*. In the script, the man in black is seen by the camera eye, yet Artaud indicates neither by whom (he uses a neutral word) nor from which camera angle or position. In the film's opening shot, the camera moves forward to a door; the following shot shows a man with his back to the camera. By placing the shots in spatial and temporal succession, the editing turns the two shots into subjective ones because of the continuity effect it creates. The appearance of the officer opening the door in the background, behind the man in black, contextualizes the look that is supposedly at the origin of the shots by integrating it into the diegesis of a sequence that has already been constituted into a story. This relationship contradicts the series of different angles that Dulac uses to show the figure of the man in black, including an extreme high-angle shot. The result is a de-diegetization of the camera's point of view as constituted in the previous shots. These incongruities justify Ivonne Allendy's criticism of Dulac:

> Mme Dulac worked single-handedly in the studio without any indications from the author; she has systematically and repeatedly forbidden him to be present at the film's editing process—a crucial one which, had it been done under the scriptwriter's supervision, would have prevented [the film's several] blunders . . . , images whose meaning is disfigured and which have only a worthless technical significance. (Quoted in Artaud, 1972)

Indeed, Dulac seems to have a sort of manneristic taste in the composition of the shots and in her use of the camera, which somehow suspends the functional value present in Artaud's script. Another incongruity, similar to the one we have just commented upon, can also be found in the opening sequence. Artaud writes: "The whole room trembles. The lamps flicker and in each trembling reflection gleams a sabre point," and in the film the flickering of the lamps is transferred onto and assumed by the camera itself. This swinging movement deforms the take, thus transferring the effect from what is looked at to the eye that is supposedly looking.

The confessional booth sequence accounts for a different effect, even though based on a similar presupposition. It is structured through a musical, rather than a discursive, editing: the melody is the focus, not the tone. According to Artaud, the face of the officer/priest is different depending on whether the person who sees him is a woman (in which case his face is sweet and pleasant) or a man (in which case his face is hard and bitter). Dulac is more concerned with the individual images than with the functional process they structure through the editing. Consequently, the hallucinogenic effect disappears, and what we have left is an accumulative succession of shots that do not follow the logic that the shot/countershot presuppose. Besides, Alex Allin's overdone gesticulation as he plays the part of the clergyman naturalizes and narrativizes the sequence, thus eliminating the poetic impact sought by Artaud.

These are not the only cases in which Dulac's interpretation of the script seems to weaken Artaud's original proposal. Let us analyze one more example. The clergyman's chase of the officer and the woman is presented in the film by means of an excessively long series of shots that break the temporal logic to which the sequence submits itself in accordance with the narrative pattern the film itself had constituted. When the officer enters the confessional booth, we see the clergyman start his chase and walk (in a series of dissolves) through a number of streets and places before arriving at the church where the two other characters are.

The narrative structure at the base of the film's representation is less the sign of an error of interpretation on Dulac's part than the indication of an understanding of the filmic discourse that is incompatible with that of Artaud. Thus, rather than a "betrayal" of Artaud's original project, the difference between the script and the film is above all the testimony of a totally different way to understand cinema as discourse. In this sense, *The Seashell and the Clergyman* is in line with Dulac's own previous and subsequent trajectory as a filmmaker. Sandy Flitterman-Lewis (1986) points to two basic notions crucial for an understanding of Dulac's work: (1) her tendency to create a "pure" kind of cinema, one closer to music than to the traditional arts; and (2) her symbolist formation.

Dulac approached the relationship between music and cinema more than once:

The cinema can certainly tell a story, but one mustn't forget that the story is nothing. The story is a surface . . . visual impact is ephemeral, it's an impact you receive which suggests a thousand thoughts. An impact analogous to that provoked by musical harmonies. (Dulac, 1928: 78; quoted in Flitterman-Lewis, 1986)

Music . . . plays with sounds in movement just as we play with images in movement . . . It is not the external fact which is really interesting, it is the emanation from within, a certain movement of things and people, viewed through the state of the soul. (Dulac, 1978: 41–42)

Consequently, Dulac believes in the power of the purely visual to create a narrative flow. According to her formulation, this flow constitutes a structure by means of an inner logic based on formal relationships and harmonies that images evoke in the viewer by triggering a series of emotional associations. She does not seem to question or investigate the historical and cultural matrix of such logic, its status as a "construct." On the contrary, its unquestioned status as a "natural" fact is in line with its capability to affect viewers who are also defined on the basis of an ambiguous and rather evanescent notion of "human nature," and whose sensorial abilities this logic stimulates by means of its evocative power. It is here where the second notion pointed out by Flitterman-Lewis becomes relevant. As an artist brought up within the symbolist tradition, Dulac is less concerned with creating structures than atmospheres. Poetic evocation was meant to affect a viewer conceived of as a passive receptor of effects and as stimulated by sensorial and/or emotional strategies. Artaud, however, conceived of the viewer as an active element forced to take active part in the sense-making process; the viewer becomes part of this process with the awareness that what constitutes the core of the aesthetic experience is not the work of the artist, but this very process itself. The question is not how to "awaken" preexisting relationships, how to constitute them or how to call meanings into being, but how to make sense. The former is a question of aesthetics; the latter is a question of how to provoke to action. The pivotal points and stakes of the two notions are quite different. This is why Dulac's and Artaud's *Seashells* are incompatible and irreconcilable projects. Dulac conceived of the film as the representation of dreamlike images; Artaud wanted to create in the viewer an effect similar to that of dreams, without reproducing the irrationality of dreams. Artaud's words of public disagreement about the film, which he wrote even before the premiere, originated precisely from this issue. Ivonne Allendy had published a brief preface to Artaud's article "Le cinéma et l'abstraction" in which she stated that *The Seashell* was "a script written from one dream." Dulac had thought of including both her own and Artaud's names as the authors of the project in the following manner: "A dream by Antonin Artaud. Visual composition by Germaine Dulac." The scriptwriter's immediate and virulent reaction led to a change to the more neutral: "Script by Antonin Artaud. Directed by Germaine Dulac." The complete script was published shortly afterward and Artaud attached to it an introduction in which he clarified his position regarding the controversy: "My script is not the representation of a dream and should not be considered as such."

Artaud and Buñuel do agree on this particular point: they do not confuse the similarity of the effects with the mechanisms producing such effects. In Dulac's notion of cinema, as we have seen, the filmic object as such is the most important element. Only as a secondary factor in the process does she approach the viewer as a whole and modifiable entity. She conceives of the logic of the unconscious that the film stimulates in the viewer as the result of a vague notion of "human nature" present in every individual in front of a screen, not as resulting from a history-specific construction. In other words, this logic ignores — or at least does not face — the fact of being itself a norm that has already been determined institutionally and internalized as a pattern, whether for behaviors, value judgments, the establishment of relational systems, and so on. Even though with apparently different goals, Dulac's film reproduces in an inverse way the functioning of the institutional mode of representation. In this sense we can define *The Seashell and the Clergyman* in terms of a "vanguardist" film.

In Artaud and Buñuel, the point of inflection has moved from the "film" as textual object to the cinematic apparatus, and therefore the notion of spectatorship changes substantially. Now the question is no longer how to address a formalized viewer sitting in the dark of the movie theater and passively waiting to react to the object's emotional stimuli in order to reconstruct a meaning perfectly inscribed by the object.[4] Instead, the question is how to conceive of the viewer as an integral and fundamental part of the filmic process as such, as an open space that is socially articulate and yet discursively deconstructable; the viewer takes active part in the events on the screen, constructs the sense of the film, and at the same time is constructed as a subject by that very process of sense construction/production.

A lot has been written about how much Buñuel's first two films owe to *The Seashell and the Clergyman*. Artaud stated something to this effect in his letter to Ivonne Allendy dated November 1929:

I feel that these people are particularly worried since *they all admit* (I have been told) the connection between *The Shell* and *Un Chien andalou* and this connection weighs heavily on them. (Artaud, 1972, 3:140; emphasis in the original)

In his letter to Jean Paulhan dated 22 January 1932, in which he expresses his most negative judgment on some of the works he considered to have imitated *The Seashell and the Clergyman*, Artaud refers to *The Age of Gold*:

This old quarrel between the surrealists and Cocteau is absurd. Because basically it is all so similar, and I assure you that people who do not know about their animal bickering put a film like *L'Age d'Or* and a film like *The Blood of a Poet* in the same sack, the one as gratuitous and useless as the other. Cocteau has been very kind to me and I will not say what I think of his film in public, at least not at the moment. — So I beg of you, in all friendship, keep this all strictly to yourself. It is secret. — But of all these films I think that *The Shell and the Clergyman* has had children, and that they are all in the same spiritual tone, but what was of interest in 1927 — because *The Shell* was a precursor — is of none in 1932, or five years later. (Artaud, 1972, 3:206–7)

In both of these letters, Artaud does not refer to the film of *The Seashell* as "his" film project. First, because 1927 is the year the script was written (the film's premiere took place in the winter of 1928). Second, because what was interesting about the first date he mentioned was his "project for a film," not the film as directed and edited by Dulac. As we have already seen, Dulac's film was interesting and new only at a superficial level, full as it was of a technical brightness as gratuitous as it was useless, as Artaud had thought.

I shall not deal in the present context with *The Age of Gold* or with its overestimated success and more conventional or, rather, vanguardist nature. Yet it is important to wonder about the extent to which Artaud was in the right when he claimed the relationship between *The Seashell* and *Un Chien andalou*.

In the chapter of their book on surrealism titled "Do Justice to Artaud," Alain and Odette Virmaux (1976) state that

a careful study of *The Seashell and the Clergyman* will prove that *Un Chien andalou* does not add much to the spirit of its time, and that it is in *The Age of Gold* that Buñuel's originality will be found.

This opinion, shared by many scholars of surrealism, implies an identification of Artaud's and Dulac's *Seashells*. At the same time it understands both

Dulac's film and *Un Chien andalou* as closured filmic texts, rather than conceiving of them in terms of cinematic apparatuses.

Therefore, it should be made clear that the establishment of a relationship between Artaud and Buñuel implies the comparison of two films, not of a film and a script. If we keep this in mind, we shall understand why Artaud thought that Buñuel had carried out part of his own project with the making of *Un Chien andalou*. And this does not mean that a real relationship should be established between Buñuel's film and Dulac's. Because Artaud's project has not been resolved cinematographically, *The Seashell* cannot constitute a reference point for Buñuel, whose most original contribution does not reside in the film's script but in the script's translation into a cinematic representation. Also in this respect, however, the similarities between Artaud's script and Buñuel's film hardly reach beyond a vaguely shared horizon.

Artaud's objective seems to affect the viewer's physicalness. Thus we have his insistence on the optical "shock," a sort of physiological "bursting" that grounds "the very act of looking." Buñuel also seems interested in the spectator's physicalness, yet with him the viewer seems to be conceived of as a position, that is, as a discursive structure; hence the relationships his film establishes with the viewer—through the film's materiality—are not based on a purely bodily dimension, but rather on an exquisitely cultural one. This means that the viewer *Un Chien andalou* addresses is not a body but a subject without physical substance, which exists as a discursive construct, and this is the reason why Artaud's project and Buñuel's in *Un Chien andalou* do not and cannot be made to coincide. Both use the technique of "free association" prompted by Breton while departing from Breton's indications in their being less interested in the production of images that would "freeze" an unconscious state than on the analysis of the effect implied by such images and their process of production. In Artaud, such analysis does not seem to find a space in which to be carried out. The literary language of the script does not give indications for the shooting process, nor does it suggest strategies that could constitute a formal alternative to Dulac's interpretation. Even though we do know that Artaud did not mean to "translate" words into images (as the director did), any attempt to come to terms with the problems posed by or in the script cannot go beyond mere hypothesis. In the case of Buñuel, however, we do have specific solutions to specific problems, based on a rigorous work of editing. The "conscious hallucination" mentioned by Goudal is no longer a "state" in which the viewer is cast; it is rather the result of a rhetorical construction that can be explained and analyzed.

Therefore, *Un Chien andalou* does not present us with the search for an aesthetic dimension of art, for what Buñuel means to question is the very notion of art as institutionalized discourse. Because of its status as mass medium, cinema allows a much better approach to this problem than literature by explicitly undermining the centrality of the speaking subject and allowing the emergence—through the editing as subject of discourse—of the impersonal narrating voice of traditional discourse as a rhetorical effect, not as the inscription-representation of a supposedly individual object. It is here where we could inscribe—in obvious disagreement with the quotation from Alain and Odette Virmaux—the "originality" of Buñuel's first film as compared to Artaud's script. *Un Chien andalou* does not deny the dominant mode of representation; it subverts its working from the inside of its established logic while pretending to be submitted by it. This is what makes *Un Chien andalou* a concrete alternative to what is in the script of *The Seashell* only a (poetic) working hypothesis.

To state that both Artaud's and Buñuel's texts are surrealist would be too hasty a judgment. First, this implies that surrealism is granted a pragmatic function that it never had, or, better said, never carried out. Second, we would confuse the well-thought-out logic of Buñuel's work and Artaud's script—if we assume that the two texts are connected conceptually—with the formal style that makes them subsumable to the theoretical postulates of the surrealists. I have already mentioned that Buñuel's public embracing of surrealism in the epigraph that introduced the film's script should be understood by taking into account the context in which it was formulated. To be accepted as a legitimate member of the surrealist group implied the endorsement of texts like that. This does not mean, however, that *Un Chien andalou* itself is to be considered as a concretion of such principles. We have already seen how the film's "poetic balance" is not just an "accident," or an uttermost resistance; rather, it is the result of a specific and very rigorously planned editing. Disorder, as Beckett would say, is part of this work not as a sort of external strategy for making sense, but because it is the truth. Let us remember Artaud's words quoted as an epigraph at the beginning of this chapter:

> Not that cinema must be devoid of all human psychology, on the contrary;
> but it should give this psychology a far more live and active form, free
> from the connections which try to make our motives appear idiotic instead
> of flaunting them in their original and profound barbarity. (*The Shell and
> the Clergyman*, in Artaud, 1972, 3:20)

If Buñuel's explicit goal was to make a "desperate, passionate call to crime," and if, in order to do so, he (re)produced the "real" mechanisms of the unconscious, wouldn't it be a more appropriate and less ambiguous approach to define both projects in terms of realism? It would certainly be a type of realism that does not have much to do with the nineteenth-century model, which appropriated the term all too easily—indeed, there is hardly anything less realistic than any of Juan Valera's novels. This kind of realism does not aim at just providing images; it is interested in analyzing the rhetorical apparatus that constitutes the images historically, and it does not pretend to reproduce the exteriority offered to our perception, but rather aims to show how both this (supposed) exteriority and our sensitivity constitute each other in their dialectical relationship, and, as such, they can be deconstructed and changed.

Un Chien andalou is not an attempt to represent a sort of "pure language" freed from the dominion of reason—a sort of nostalgic reminiscing for a lost paradise. This is what determined the inscription of nostalgia in so many of the official surrealist texts.[5] Nostalgia is absent from Buñuel's works. Perhaps because of this, none of his films presents us with an idealized vision of the lower social classes. There is never the simplistic juxtaposition between an ever-evil master and the natural goodness of the exploited. His work does not represent "nature" but "culture." Both terms—the master, the exploited—are the result of the same system; both may share the same values. In a society based on the fight for survival, the very notions of evil and good do not have much sense. Thus, brutality is as much a feature of life in *Land without Bread* (remember the cockfight sequence) as of the blind man in *The Young and the Damned* or of the beggars in *Viridiana*. This harsh and merciless vision, void of any sense of false pity, was probably what caused the rejection of Buñuel's first two films at the time of their first public showings. Neither of the two provides the viewer any sort of sentimental alibi to silence and appease his or her conscience.

This standpoint is found in Buñuel not only in his filmmaking; it had been explicitly theorized in his earlier writings, before his first film, and would be present in all his works after *Un Chien andalou*, especially in the period following the making of *Land without Bread*. This latter film is a milestone in the director's trajectory: because Buñuel had total control over it (even with the later process of sonorization), the changes he introduced to the model represented by *Un Chien andalou* concerning the story's higher (or more apparent) level of intelligibility do not result from pressure from the industrial system. Rather, they arise from the director's explicit desire to make the issues clearer and more easily readable. *Land without Bread*, however, the film that closes the trilogy of what has been called Buñuel's "independent phase," retrospectively allows a different reading of his discursive proposal carried out in the previous films. In *Land without Bread* there are documentary images: they do not *represent* facts, objects, or actions; they *present* themselves as the filmic trace of a real extradiscursive material. Yet, in spite of this, we see the goat plunge from the rock, seen from a point of view that is impossible in a documentary. Shot 115 is an establishing shot showing a goat that starts to fall off the edge of an escarpment.[6] A direct cut shows an extreme high-angle close-up of the animal as it falls. It is obvious that the randomness that the "documentary" implies, its "nonrepresentational" matrix, makes it highly improbable to foresee the death of the goat in such a precise way as to place the camera at exactly the right time and place and shoot from two different angles at the same time. We do not know whether shot 116 was made after the animal's death by dropping the goat's corpse in order to film its fall, but we do know that the two shots, by fictionalizing the documentary, that is, by representing the animal's death, unmask the rhetorical nature of the effect of truth and annul the supposedly referential value of the images by moving their sense from the supposed exteriority of the discourse to the apparatus that produces it. The opposition art / reality can then no longer be approached by considering the two terms as individual and independent entities; instead, they should be understood as discursive constructs that only exist within their mutual relationship. Thus an "aesthetic" logic no longer has a meaning.

Buñuel's later films are grounded on this uninterrupted dialogue between presentation and representational effect as mobile and interchangeable terms, thus detaching his work from the surrealist model. Dalí's model for the cinematic compositional strategy, for example, consisted of a "realistic" contextualization of "surrealist" elements in order to stress, through contrast, the presence of the latter. The dialogue his paintings establish with the real landscape of Cadaqués or with themes and topics of the history of painting is based on a presupposed separateness between the two spaces, on the belief that reality—whether physical (Cadaqués) or discursive (art history as institution)—exists as separate from art and its practice. In Buñuel, this separation does not exist outside the field connecting both spaces.

This procedure was already present in *Un Chien andalou*, where the citations of Vermeer and Millet are not cultural winks to the viewer; they become meaningful thanks to the dialogue they establish through the editing with other elements of the film. We can track down their presence in Buñuel's previous literary works, as Agustín Sánchez-Vidal (1982) pointed out in his introduction to Buñuel's *Obra literaria*.

The position of the so-called poetic avant-garde of the 1920s, that is, the Generation of 1927 (with which Buñuel entailed personal relationships), implied that the radical innovation that Buñuel sought was somehow subordinated to a practice easily subsumed by the intellectual classes of dominant European liberalism, which had in Ortega y Gasset's *Revista de Occidente* its most representative exponent. Vicente Huidobro, Juan Larrea, and Pepín Bello, together with members of previous generations such as Ramón del Valle-Inclán and Ramón Gómez de la Serna, proposed alternatives that could be easily co-opted by such proposal. Buñuel's stand on this respect was always clear-cut. We have already commented on his attack of Juan Ramón Jiménez: far from being the impertinent gesture of a young man looking for a spot in the sun, it should be read from the context of Buñuel's private and public activities, in which the would-be writer exposed what was already the core of a coherent intellectual project.

In his letter to Pepín Bello dated 1 October 1928 we read the following:

> We have to fight with all the scorn and anger we possess, against all traditional poetry, from Homer and Goethe, including Góngora—the foulest monster born of a mother—right up to the ruinous debris of today's poetasters . . . You will understand the distance which separates you, Dalí and me from all our poetic friends. They are antagonistic worlds, the earth's pole and the south of Mars; and they all belong in the crater of vilest putrefaction. Federico wants to do surrealist things, but they are false, done with *intelligence*, which can never discover the things which instinct discovers. His last piece published in the *Gaceta* is an instance of his trouble. It is as artistic as his *Ode to the Blessed Sacrament* and will raise an erection in the feeble member of Falla and other Andalusian artists. In spite of everything, within the traditional context, Federico is one of the best. (Aranda, 1976, 48; also collected in Sánchez-Vidal, 1982)

Leaving aside the letter's virulent and, perhaps, unfair tone, it should be pointed out that Buñuel does not confuse value judgment with personal appreciation. He accepts whatever good there is in the traditional panorama without ceasing to consider it as such. His criticism is to be found in his rejection of bombastic, flowery forms—in short, of all that could be reduced to an easily neutralizable formalism.

Góngora's centennial was in 1927. Curiously enough, as we previously noted, Goya's centennial (1928) was celebrated one year early so as to have it coincide—and therefore somewhat compete—with Gongora's. The project of Gómez de la Serna and Buñuel about *Los caprichos*, mentioned in chapter 2, should be read in this context. It was meant to constitute a practice nonrecuperable by the classicist tradition, which was quite remote from the sub-versiveness that, in the authors' opinion, "nonartistic" art and literature should have.

If we read the poems that Buñuel included in his collection entitled *Un Chien andalou*, we will clearly see to what extent his positions in his first film are in line with this standpoint. Let us look at two examples, the poem "No me parece bien ni mal," and a fragment from "Bird of Anguish."

> I think that sometimes we are looked at
> from the front, the back and the side
> by malicious henlike eyes
> more frightful than the rotten water from the caves
> incestuous as the eyes of a mother
> sent to the gallows
> sticky as an intercourse
> like the rotten gelatin swallowed by vultures
>
> I think I will die
> with my hands sunk in the mud of country roads
>
> I believe that were I to beget a child
> he would endlessly stare
> at the animals copulating at dusk.

* * *

> A pleniosaur slept between my eyes
> As the music burnt in a lamp
> And the landscape felt a passion of Tristan and Isolde.
>
> Your body molded itself to mine
> As a hand molds to the thing it wants to hide; . . .
> All love dialogues are alike
> All have the same delirious chords . . .
> Then comes the prayer and the wind,
> The wind that weaves sounds in sharp points
> With a sweetness of blood
> Of howls, made into flesh . . . [7]

The imagery of these poems is similar to what we will later find in Rafael Alberti's *Concerning the Angels* and *Sermones y moradas*, Luis Cernuda's *Forbidden Pleasures*, or Vicente Aleixandre's *Espadas como labios* and *La destrucción o el amor*. However, neither the underlying structure that produces this imagery nor the articulation of the images as a structure are the same. There is something more deeply disturbing in Buñuel: his more virulent use of metaphors, his deliberate refusal to embellish images, which are always quite rough in their bareness, and, above all, the total disappearance of the old order of things, which is never restored to new life, never seen in a different light or upside down, as happens with the other authors.

The image of "the animals copulating at dusk" as borderless horizon for the gaze, makes of the outside world a pile of objects that are both irreducible to their referential function and deprived of all symbolic charge. Only Lorca's *Poet in New York*—which was indebted to Buñuel's proposal—would later be able to articulate a similarly critical and subversive project.

The real, radical subversiveness (an attempt not to turn the system upside down or to make it simply more comprehensive, but to deconstruct it) is to be sought in the *realism* rather than in the *surrealism* of Buñuel's and other theoreticians' projects. Both the former and the latter (Léiris, Artaud, or Bataille) had once shared the views of the Bretonian group, but soon became aware of its impasse. Thus Bataille writes in his *Théorie de la réligion* something that it is not hard to imagine Buñuel would have agreed with: "The work of the mason, who assembles, is the work that matters. Thus the adjoining bricks, in a book, should not be less visible than the new brick, which is the book. What is offered the reader, in fact, cannot be an element, but must be the ensemble in which it is inserted: it is the whole human assemblage and edifice, which must be, not just a pile of scraps, but rather a self-consciousness."[8]

Script and Description of the Découpage of *Un Chien andalou*

The original script of *Un Chien andalou* has been published many times. It appeared in *Révue du cinéma 5*, November 1929; in *La Révolution Surréaliste* 12, 1929; in *Premier Plan* 13, October 1960; in Ado Kyrou (1963); in *L'Avant-Scène du Cinéma* 27–28 (double issue), June-July 1963. It was published by Era in Mexico (Spanish version by José de la Colina) in 1971; by Verband der Deutschen Filmclubs, Bad Ems, 1965; by Lorrimer, London, 1968; by Simon and Schuster, New York, 1968; and by Einaudi, Turin, 1974. The translation published by Lorrimer is often considered the standard English version of the script.

Many differences exist between the original script and the edited film. Because the reading provided by this book is based both on the film and on the precise specifications that appear in the script (no matter whether followed or not), I have included a description of the photographic découpage presented in appendix 2. The text from the original script appears in italics. Changes and cuts introduced during the shooting are indicated in the notes.

> *The publication of this script in* La Révolution Surréaliste *is the only one I have authorized. It expresses, with no reservations whatsoever, my complete support of surrealist thought and practice.* Un Chien andalou *would not exist had surrealism not existed.*
>
> *"A successful film": this is what most of the people who saw it think about it. What can I do against buffs of every novelty, even if this novelty offends their deepest convictions, against a corrupt and insincere press, against the idiotic crowd that has found "beautiful" or "poetic" what is but a desperate, passionate call to crime?*
>
> Luis Buñuel

Credits

Producer and director: Luis Buñuel.
Script: Luis Buñuel and Salvador Dalí.
Music: Fragments from Richard Wagner's *Tristan and Isolde*, and Argentinean tangos.
Photography: Albert Dubergen (Duverger).
Setting: Pierre Schilzneck.
Editing: Luis Buñuel.
Cast: Simone Mareuil (the woman); Pierre Batcheff (the man); Jaime Miravilles, Salvador Dalí, and Luis Buñuel.
Running time: 16′ 14″
Length: 430 meters.
Silent film in black and white.

In the existing copies of the film the following text appears in transparency before the credits and scrolls up the screen in coincidence with the beginning of the tango music (tango no. 1) of the sound track.

> The sound track music is from records of La Guide Internationale du Disque. *Tristan and Isolde*, by Richard Wagner, is played by the Frankfurt Opera Orchestra, conducted by Carl Bamberger.
> The sonorization of the integral version of this film was made in 1960, following Buñuel's instructions, in accordance with the live sonorization he himself made with records during the first show.

After the credits an intertitle appears, printed in white on a black background, with the following text:

Il était une fois . . . (Once upon a time . . .)

A balcony. At night. A man is sharpening a razor by the balcony.

The sound track music changes to *Tristan and Isolde*. Fade-in to:

Shot 1. Close-up of two hands sharpening a razor by a window without curtains, lit by a diffused light. A wristwatch with a black leather band on the left forearm.

Shot 2. Camera turned 90° to the right. Close-up of a man's head looking down with a cigarette in his mouth. His eyes wink almost imperceptibly. The man wears an open striped shirt without collar, the sleeves rolled up to the elbow. The windows now have curtains.

Shot 3. The position of the camera is identical to that of shot 1. The man is still sharpening the razor; he tries its sharpness against the nail of his left thumb.

Shot 4. Same as shot 2.

Shot 5. Medium shot of the man. On the left, a window with curtains and dark drapes. Tracking shot of the man as he stops by the window, which he opens, and goes out. On the left of the frame, the window with curtains and dark drapes. The window is now shown as a French window.

Shot 6. Countershot. Medium shot of the man going out to the balcony and leaning against the railing. We can see the wrought-iron railing and the plants on the balcony.

The man looks through a window at the sky and sees . . .
A light cloud passing across the face of the full moon.

Shot 7. Camera turned 135° to the right. Close-up of the man looking up to the off-screen space on the right of the frame.

Shot 8. Countershot. A dark sky and a full moon on the left of the frame. A narrow, long white cloud moves toward the moon from the left.

Shot 9. Continuation of the end of shot 7.

Then the head of a young woman with wide-open eyes. The blade of the razor moves toward one of her eyes. The light cloud now moves across the face of the moon. The razor blade slits the eye of the young woman, dividing it.

Shot 10. Close-up of a woman's face. A man's left hand stretches open her left eye by pressing his thumb on her eyebrow and his forefinger under her lower eyelid. He wears the same shirt as the man in the previous shots, but also a necktie with diagonal stripes, and he does not wear a wristwatch. The man's right hand holds a razor in front of the woman's face. He starts a movement from the right to the left of the frame.

Shot   11.   Cut to a shot of the cloud moving across the moon.

Shot   12.   Close-up of an eye whose pupil is slit by a razor. The fluid from the eye oozes out. Short fade and cut to an intertitle that says:

Huit ans après. (Eight years later.)

A deserted road. It is raining.[1] *A man, dressed in a dark-gray suit and riding a bicycle, appears. The man's head, back, and waist are decked in white frills. A rectangular box with black and white diagonal stripes hangs from a thong on his chest. The man's feet pedal automatically and he is not holding the handlebars: his hands are resting on his knees. Medium shot of him seen from behind, then shot of him superimposed on shot of the street, down which he is cycling with his back to camera.*

Shot   13.   Tango no. 2 starts playing. Long shot of a deserted street with high buildings on both sides. The sun is shining. A figure on a bicycle, seen from behind, enters the frame, biking along the street toward the background.

Shot   14.   Camera turned 145° to the left. Long shot of the cyclist moving towards the left of the frame.

He cycles toward camera until the striped box fills the screen.

Shot   15.   Dissolve to a close-up of the cyclist moving toward the camera. He is a young man. His head, waist, and shoulders are covered by white frills. He wears a collar and a dark necktie. A little box with black and white diagonal stripes hangs from his neck.

Shot   16.   Tracking shot from the bicycle. Long subjective shot of the street; a crowd starts to gather in the background.

Shot   17.   Camera turned 180°. The cyclist moves toward the camera. In the foreground we can clearly see the box hanging from a strap over his chest.

Shot   18.   Continuation of shot 16.

Shot   19.   Dissolve to a medium shot of the cyclist seen from the back. Fade-out, then fade-in to a reverse angle shot of the street.

Shot   20.   Long shot of the cyclist moving from the left toward the camera.

Shot 21.   Dissolve to a close-up of the box.

A room on the third floor of a building overlooking the street. A young woman in a brightly colored dress is sitting in the center of the room; she is absorbed in reading a book.

Shot 22.   Tango no. 2 stops and the music from *Tristan and Isolde* starts playing. Fade-in to a long shot of a room. In the background are a bedside table with a lamp, and a bed on the left. At the center is a French window similar to the one in shot 5. A woman sits in the middle of the room, facing a table and with her back to the bed; she is attentively reading a book.

She gives a start,

Shot 23.   Dissolve to a medium medium low-angle shot of the woman. She seems to be the same woman of the initial sequence; she wears the same clothes. The woman remains on the left of the frame. She reads. Suddenly startled, she looks up.

Shot 24.   Long shot of the cyclist moving from the left to the right of the frame.

listens for something and throws the book onto a nearby couch.

Shot 25.   Continuation of shot 23 in medium shot. The woman, seemingly startled, hurls the book on a sofa.

The book remains opened to a reproduction of Vermeer's "The Lacemaker."

Shot 26.   Close-up of the book, showing a reproduction of Vermeer's *The Lacemaker.*

The young woman is now convinced that something interesting is taking place; she gets up, half-turns, and walks quickly over to the window.

Shot 27.   Long medium shot of the woman getting up and walking offscreen at the right of the frame.

Shot 28.   Long medium shot of the woman—shown in reverse shot—

moving from the right to the left of the frame. She stops by the window and looks outside.

The cyclist has just stopped, below in the street.

Shot   29.   Long high-angle tracking shot of the cyclist moving from the upper right angle to the lower middle part of the frame. A gaslight is at the right of the frame.

Out of sheer inertia, without trying to keep his balance, he topples over into the muddy gutter.[2]

Shot   30.   Continuation of shot 28. The woman, startled or scared by what she sees, closes the curtains and steps back.

Shot   31.   Continuation of shot 29, with the camera turned slightly to the left of the frame. The bicycle stops, the young man loses his balance and falls sideways on the edge of the sidewalk at his left.

Shot   32.   Long medium shot of the woman with her back to the window, her arms akimbo and a pensive expression on her face. Suddenly she turns to the window and looks outside.

Shot   33.   Camera turned 180°. Long high-angle shot of the man on the ground, with part of his body on the sidewalk and the bicycle wheels turning aimlessly.

Shot   34.   Continuation of shot 32.

Shot   35.   Long shot of the woman with her back to the window. In the middle, the table with the open book. On the left, a bedside table with a lamp and the bed. The woman moves toward the bed.

The young woman, looking resentful and outraged, dashes out of the room and down the stairs.

Shot   36.   A long medium shot continues the previous shot through a *raccord* in the movement. The woman moves to the left, reaches the door, opens it, and goes out.

Close-up of the cyclist lying on the ground, expressionless, in exactly the same position as when he fell.[3]

Shot   37.   Close-up of the man on the ground stretched diagonally, with his feet in the lower left and the head in the upper right of the frame. Now all his body lies on the street, with only his left temple on the sidewalk edge. He winks faintly.

The young woman runs out of the house toward him and throws herself on him to kiss him passionately on the lips, the eyes, and the nose. It is now raining so hard that the rain blots out what is happening on screen.[4]

Shot   38.   Long shot of the woman going out of the room and down the stairs toward the lower part of the frame, through which she disappears.

Shot   39.   Medium shot of the fallen man. The camera is in the same position as in shot 37, yet the man lies face up now, with his nape on the edge of the sidewalk. In the middle part of the frame we can clearly see the striped box on his chest.

Shot   40.   Long medium shot of the woman going out of the front door. She wrings her hands nervously and moves to the lower left part of the frame.

Shot   41.   Medium shot of the woman holding the head of the fallen man in her hands. She kisses him repeatedly and passionately.

Dissolve to the box: its diagonal stripes are superimposed on the diagonal lines of falling rain. Hands holding a little key open the box and pull out a tie wrapped in striped tissue paper. The rain, the box, the tissue paper, and the tie make up a pattern of diagonal stripes of varying sizes.

Shot   42.   Dissolve to a close-up of the box. The woman's right hand, with an oval-shaped ring on her ring finger, inserts a key in the lock. She opens the box. Inside the box is a paper wrapping with black diagonal stripes on a white background.

The same room. The young woman is standing by the bed, looking at the various items worn by the cyclist—frilly cuffs, box, starched collar, and plain black tie. All these things are laid out on the bed as though they were being worn by someone lying on the bed. The young woman finally decides to reach out, and she picks up the collar, removes the plain tie from it, and puts in its place the striped tie that she has just taken out of the box. She then puts the collar back where it was and sits down by the bed like someone at a vigil. The blanket and pillow on the bed are slightly rumpled as though a body really were lying there.[5]

Shot 43.   Medium shot of the woman on the right of the frame leaning over a bed. She opens the paper wrapping and uncovers a necktie with diagonal stripes of equal width, and a starched collar. She wraps the necktie around the collar.

Shot 44.   Close-up of the bed where white frills are laid. The woman wraps the necktie around the collar and places both on the upper frills. Backward tracking shot. Beneath the necktie we see the locked box and the frills that covered the cyclist's hips.

Shot 45.   Medium shot of the woman moving around the bed; she sits down and stares at the bed with her back to the camera.

Shot 46.   Long shot of the bed with all the pieces placed in an orderly way on the bedspread. The collar closes and the necktie, which now has a knot, seems to surround an invisible neck.

Shot 47.   Medium low-angle shot of the woman sitting and looking toward the left side of the frame.

Shot 48.   Same as shot 46; now the closing of the collar and the necktie are shown not by means of a cut but through a dissolve.

The young woman seems to be aware of someone standing behind her and she turns to see who it is. Without showing any surprise, she sees that it is the same man, no longer wearing any of the items that are laid out on the bed. He is looking at something on his right palm with great concentration and some distress.

Shot 49.   Close-up of the woman's face looking as pensive as in shot 47. She suddenly raises her head and turns to the upper right of the frame.

Shot 50.   Medium shot of the cyclist, his hair slightly in disorder, standing sideways to the camera with his left hand on his hip on the right-hand side of the frame. He wears a gray double-breasted suit. He stares at his right hand. A door is on the left of the frame.

The young woman goes over to him and also looks at what he has in his hand. Close-up of the hand full of ants crawling out of a black hole in the palm. None of the ants falls off.

Shot 51.   Close-up of the man's hand. Ants are swarming on his palm. They come out of a hole in the middle of his palm.

Shot 52.   Same as shot 50.

Shot 53.   Medium shot of the woman in an expectant attitude. She leans against the back of a chair, looking toward the right, then she gets up.

Shot 54.   Long shot of the room. The woman, with her back to the camera, leaves the chair and moves toward the man, who is still staring at his right hand.

Shot 55.   Camera turned 135°. Medium shot of both the man and the woman staring at the man's hand. The man wears an unbuttoned shirt and no necktie.

Shot 56.   Close-up of the hand with the ants.

Shot 57.   Same camera position as in shot 55. The woman looks at the man, the man looks at the woman; the woman looks at the hand, the man does the same.

Shot 58.   Same as shot 56.

Dissolve to the hairs on the armpit of a young woman who is lying on a beach in the sunshine. Dissolve to the undulating spines of a sea urchin.[6] Dissolve to the head of a young woman seen directly from above. This shot is taken as though through the iris of an eye: the iris opens to reveal a group of people standing around the young woman and trying to push their way through a police barrier.

Shot 59.   Dissolve to a close-up of someone's right armpit—seemingly a woman wearing a swimsuit, and hiding her face with a hat.

Shot 60.   Dissolve to a sea urchin, motionless in the lower middle of the frame.

Shot 61.   Dissolve to a long, high-angle iris shot (with the iris half-closed) of someone poking with a stick at a severed hand lying on the ground.

Shot 62.   Same as previous shot, but with the camera closer to the figure with the stick, in medium shot.

In the middle of the circle, the young woman is using a stick to try to pick up a severed hand with painted fingernails that is lying on the ground.[7] A policeman goes up to her and begins rebuking her. He leans down, picks up the hand, wraps it up carefully, and puts it inside the striped box that had been hanging around the cyclist's neck. He hands the box over to the young woman; she thanks him and he salutes.[8]
As the policeman gives her the box, she seems to be completely carried away by a strange emotion and is oblivious of everything that is going on around her. It is as though she were listening to some distant religious music, perhaps music she heard when she was a child.

Shot 63.   The beginning of this shot is the same as the beginning of shot 61. Iris-in to a group of people surrounding the person poking at the severed hand. Behind this person is a man wearing a police hat.

Shot 64.   Camera turned 45°. Two policemen push back the crowd surrounding the person poking at the hand, who is now standing sideways to the camera in a slight high-angle shot.

Shot 65.   Camera turned 90° in the same direction. Medium shot of the person looking at the lower right part of the frame. It is a girl dressed in a suit and with a masculine-looking hairstyle. She wears a plain dark necktie.

Shot 66.   Close-up of the severed hand lying diagonally on the ground, from the lower right to the upper left side, on a rough surface. Someone is poking at it with a stick coming down from the upper left side of the frame.

Shot 67.   Medium shot of the crowd getting closer. The police push them back.

Shot 68.   Same as shot 65.

Shot 69.   Medium shot of the crowd looking. A policeman moves from the right to the left of the frame with his back to the camera, and disappears.

Shot 70.   Close-up of the crowd looking. One of the onlookers, who wears a gray suit and has a handkerchief in the upper pocket of his double-breasted jacket, has a fearful expression on his face as he holds tightly his left wrist with his right hand.

Shot 71. Medium medium high-angle shot of the girl's hand, legs, and stick. The position of the camera is the same as in shot 65.

Shot 72. Medium high-angle close-up of the onlooking crowd. In the middle is a woman wearing a hat and a suit with a collar bordered with lace.

Shot 73. Medium medium low-angle shot of the woman and the man from the sequence in the room, looking from the window with the half-open curtains. The man moves his head to his right.

Shot 74. Same as shot 65.

Shot 75. Same as beginning of shot 73.

Shot 76. Long medium shot (medium low-angle) of the young woman in the middle part of the frame surrounded by the crowd; a policeman on the left of the frame looks to the offscreen space on the left. The policeman turns, moves toward the young girl, and greets her in a military manner, by raising his right hand to his hat.

Shot 77. Medium shot of the policeman speaking with the girl as he points to something offscreen below them both (presumably the severed hand).

Shot 78. Long high-angle shot of the policeman bending to pick up the severed hand. The girl remains motionless.

Shot 79. Camera in the same position as in shot 77. Medium shot of the policeman placing the severed hand in a box. When he closes the box, we see that its cover has diagonal black and white stripes.

The crowd's curiosity has died down. People are moving off in all directions. The couple has been looking at the scene from behind the window on the third floor all this time. We can see them through the window, from which we too have been watching the end of the scene. When the policeman gives the box to the young woman, the two people in the room also seem overwhelmed with the same emotion. They nod as though in rhythm to that dis-

tant music that only the young woman can hear.[9] *The man looks at the woman and makes a gesture as though to say, "You see? Didn't I tell you?"*

Shot 80.   Medium shot of the young woman on the street looking at the left-hand side of the frame. She picks up the box and holds it against her chest.

Shot 81.   Low-angle close-up of the woman and the man looking outside through the window pane. The man looks up in the distance.

Shot 82.   Same as shot 80.

Shot 83.   Same as shot 81. Now the woman too looks up in the distance.

Shot 84.   Long shot of the girl in the street with the box in her hands, the policeman talking to her, and the crowd around them. The policeman disperses the crowd. They all move offscreen; only the girl remains in the frame.

She looks down at the street again, where the young woman, all alone now, stands as if rooted to the spot, incapable of moving, as cars drive past her at great speed. Suddenly one of the cars runs her over and leaves her lying in the street, horribly mangled.[10]

Shot 85.   Camera turned 135°. Medium shot of the girl holding the box against her chest. Now she wears a long gray overcoat, a shirt, and a necktie with black and white diagonal stripes. A car moves from the lower left to the upper right of the frame behind her.

Shot 86.   Insert of close-up of the man looking lustfully outside the window.

Shot 87.   End of shot 85.

Shot 88.   Medium shot of the man and the woman in the room. The man looks at the woman with desire as he leans with his left elbow against the window with closed curtains. The woman, with her back to the camera, looks outside through the curtains.

Shot 89.   Camera in the same position as in shot 84, turned 45° to the left. Long high-angle shot of the young woman in the street. A car moves from the lower to the upper right of the frame and disappears.

Shot 90.   Same as shot 86.

Shot 91. Same as shot 89.

Shot 92. Medium shot of the girl in the street holding the box against her chest as she looks to the right-hand side of the frame. Camera turned 90° as compared to shot 85. A shadow moves from the left- to the right-hand side of the frame in the foreground.

Shot 93. Long shot of a car moving straight-on toward the camera.

Shot 94. Same as shot 92.

Shot 95. Long tracking shot from inside the car moving toward the girl. She has an expression of terror on her face and hurls her hand up. The box lies on the ground by her feet.

Shot 96. Same as shot 94. The girl moves in fear, pressing the box against her chest.

Shot 97. Medium shot of the girl as the car moves toward her. The car runs her down.

Shot 98. Same as shot 86.

Shot 99. Long high-angle shot of the girl lying face up on the ground in the lower right part of the frame. We can see the box lying above her left arm. The car disappears on the upper left side of the frame. Several people enter the frame and move toward the body on the ground.

The man, with the determination of someone who feels sure of his rights, goes over to the young woman and, after staring at her lustfully with rolling eyes, grabs her breasts through her dress. Close-up of the man's hands fondling the breasts, which appear through the dress. The man's face has a terrible look, almost of mortal anguish, and a stream of blood-flecked saliva begins to run out of the corner of his mouth onto the naked breasts.[11] The breasts disappear to become a pair of thighs, which the man kneads.[12] His expression has changed. His eyes now shine with cruelty and lust. His mouth, which was wide open, now puckers up like an anus.

Shot 100. Same as shot 86. At the end of the shot the man turns to the right.

Shot 101. Medium shot of the woman and the man (with his back to the camera) in the room by the window, with closed curtains.

Shot 102.   Same frame composition as in shot 101, with the camera turned 135° to the right.

Shot 103.   Same as shot 101. The woman looks in fear at the man.

Shot 104.   Same as shot 102. The man looks lustfully at the woman's body as he leans nonchalantly against the window crossbar.

Shot 105.   Camera turned 45° to the left. Medium shot of the man looking lustfully at the woman; he gets closer to her and attempts to fondle her breasts. The music from *Tristan and Isolde* stops. She pushes him away.

Shot 106.   Medium shot of the man moving from the left- to the right-hand side of the frame. At this moment tango music (no. 1) starts playing again in the sound track. From here to shot 111 the man's movements seem to follow the rhythm of the tango music.

Shot 107.   Countershot. Medium shot of the woman stepping back.

Shot 108.   Continuation of shot 106.

Shot 109.   Continuation of shot 107. The man enters the frame from the left, gets near the woman, and attempts to push her against the wall. She pushes him away. He finally places his hands on her breasts.

Shot 110.   Close-up of the man's hands fondling the woman's breasts. The woman attempts to push his hands away.

Shot 111.   Medium shot of the woman, who finally manages to get rid of the man's hold. He tries again, and this time she does not resist.

Shot 112.   Same as shot 110, with the camera turned 45° to the left.

Shot 113.   Dissolve to a close-up of the man's hands caressing a woman's naked breasts.

Shot 114.   Low-angle close-up of the man's face with the eyes rolled to the back of his head, his head up as he salivates.

Shot 115.   Same as shot 113, with the camera slightly turned to the right.

Shot 116.   Dissolve to a close-up of the man's hands fondling the woman's breasts through her dress.

Shot 117.   Same as shot 114.

Shot 118.   Medium close-up of the man's hands fondling the woman's breasts through her dress.

Shot 119.   Dissolve to a close-up of two hands fondling two naked buttocks.

Shot 120.   Dissolve to medium close-up of the man's hands.

Shot 121.   Close-up of the man gaping at the woman, part of whose head appears in the lower right of the frame.

The young woman moves back toward the middle of the room, followed by the man, still in the same state.

She suddenly breaks his hold on her and escapes from his grasp.[13]

The man's mouth tightens with anger. The young woman realizes that a really disagreeable and violent scene is about to take place. She inches away until she reaches a corner of the room, where she crouches behind a little table.[14]

Shot 122.   Same as end of shot 111. The woman pushes the man away.

Shot 123.   Long shot of the woman running around the table and toward the bed; the man runs after her.

Shot 124.   Long shot of the woman jumping over the bed. The camera tracks behind her until she reaches the window, then pans to the man who moves in exactly the same way as the woman. The camera tracks backward to show the man and the woman as she crouches in a corner behind a chair and he stands in an expectant attitude.

Shot 125.   Medium shot of the woman picking up a tennis racket from the wall and lifting it in order to protect herself.

The man, now looking like the villain in a melodrama, looks around, trying to find something. He sees a piece of rope lying on the floor and picks it up with his right hand. He then gropes about with his left hand and picks up another identical piece of rope.

The young woman, glued to the wall, looks with horror at what her aggressor is doing.[15]

The man begins advancing toward her, pulling at the rope and making a great effort to drag whatever is attached to the ropes.

Shot 126.   Over-the-shoulder long shot from behind the man with the camera in the same position as in the previous shot. The man turns and looks down; he seems to be looking for something.

Shot 127.   Medium shot of the man with a sadistic sneer on his face.

Shot 128.   Same as shot 125.

Shot 129.   Same as shot 127.

Shot 130.   Medium shot of the woman raising the tennis racket with a menacing expression on her face.

Shot 131.   Same as shot 129. The man's expression changes from sadism to amazement.

Shot 132.   Same as shot 130. The woman has a gesture of contempt.

Shot 133.   Same as shot 131. The man starts searching his pockets. He suddenly looks down and smiles at the woman with an expression of satisfaction on his face.

Shot 134.   Medium medium high-angle shot of the man crouching on the floor as he picks up the ends of a rope.

Shot 135.   Same as shot 132. The woman has an expression of amazement and fear on her face.

First we see a cork, then a melon, then two Brothers of Christian Schools, then finally, two magnificent grand pianos containing the carcasses of two donkeys. Their feet, tails, rumps, and excrement are spilling out of the lids. As one of the grand pianos is pulled past the camera, we can see the big head of one of the donkeys hanging down over the keyboard. The man pulls at this with great difficulty, straining desperately toward the young woman, knocking over chairs, tables, a standing lamp, and other objects in his path. The rumps of the donkeys get caught in everything. A stripped bone hits the light hanging from the ceiling, so that it rocks from side to side until the end of the scene.[16]

Shot 136.   Long shot of the man dragging something with the ropes as the woman looks at him in amazement; he falls, gets up, and pulls with all his might. Two rectangular corkboards are attached to the ropes.

Shot 137. Medium shot of the man entering the frame from the right as he pulls at the ropes with great effort.

Shot 138. Same as shot 135. The woman drops the tennis racket.

Shot 139. Continuation of shot 137.

Shot 140. Camera turned 90° to the right. Long shot of the room. The woman drops the tennis racket (*raccord* in the movement with shot 138). The man, seen from the back, drags a Marist brother with each rope, and a grand piano with a dead donkey on top.

Shot 141. Close-up of the head of the dead donkey hanging down over the piano keyboard.

Shot 142. Same as shot 140. Tango no. 1 ends.

Shot 143. Medium shot of the woman attempting to step back; she cannot, and hides her face in the corner with a fearful gesture.

Shot 144. Same as shot 139. Tango no. 2 begins in the middle of the shot.

Shot 145. Close-up of the two Marist brothers being dragged from the left to the right of the frame. They wear their religious outfit: black cassock with a sash around the waist, a wide-brimmed black hat, and a starched white collar on the chest.

Shot 146. Camera turned 90° to the right. Long high-angle shot of the man pulling the two Marist brothers.

Shot 147. Close-up of the woman in the corner as she turns her face to the camera with a fearful expression.

Shot 148. Same as shot 141.

Shot 149. Same as shot 145. A different actor plays the part of the Marist brother on the right.

Shot 150. Same as shot 146.

Shot 151. Same as shot 142.

Shot 152. Same as shot 144. From the left of the frame the woman looks in amazement at the man.

When the man is just about to reach the young woman, she rushes out of the room. Her attacker lets go of the ropes and hurls himself after her. The young woman manages to get out of the room into the next one, but not quickly enough to slam the door shut. The man's hand is trapped in the door, caught in the jamb.[17]

Shot 153.   Close-up of the woman with an expression of amazement on her face. She looks at her left, starts to run, and disappears from the frame.

Shot 154.   Medium shot of the woman opening the door and exiting the room. The man drops the ropes and runs after her.

Shot 155.   Close-up of the man attempting to get to the door; the door closes on his arm, preventing him from going out.

Shot 156.   Countershot. Close-up of the woman pushing the door to prevent the man from opening it.

Shot 157.   Long medium shot of the man, his face to the camera, leaning against the wall with his arm caught in the door and an expression of pain on his face.

Shot 158.   Close-up of the man with an expression of pain on his face, his right hand on his head and his left arm caught in the door.

Shot 159.   Same as shot 156.

Shot 160.   Close-up of the woman looking at a hand, caught in the door, with ants swarming on its palm. (A hand is now caught in the door instead of an arm.)

Shot 161.   Close-up of the hand with the swarming ants.

Shot 162.   Same as shot 158.

Shot 163.   Same as shot 161. The hand clenches in a fist.

Shot 164.   Same as shot 159.

In the other room, the young woman pushes harder and harder at the door, watching the fingers of the hand moving painfully and slowly as the ants begin crawling out of the palm onto the door.[18] *The young woman turns away to look at the room, which is identical to the previous one except that different lighting gives it a different appearance: the young woman sees . . .*

The same bed is there, with the same man lying on it, the one who has still got his hand in the door. He is wearing the frills, and the box lies on his chest. He does not move at all, but stares with wide-open eyes that seem to be saying, "Something really extraordinary is just about to happen!"

Shot 165. Long shot of the man lying on the bed. The lamp is lit. He wears the white frills the cyclist was wearing at the beginning of the film, and the necktie that was in the box (see shot 43). The striped box is placed on his chest.

Shot 166. Camera turned 135° to the right. Close-up of the man lying in bed, his head on the pillow.

Shot 167. Same as shot 164. The woman, surprised by what she sees on the right-hand side of the frame, stops pushing the door with her body.

Shot 168. Same as shot 166. The man rolls his eyes to the left of the frame and smiles with an evil expression.

Shot 169. Same as shot 167.

Shot 170. Same as shot 168.

The following words appear on a black screen:

Vers trois heures du matin. (About 3 A.M.)

A stranger, seen from behind, is stopping on the landing outside the apartment. He rings the bell. Unlike in other silent films of the period,[19] we do not see the actual electric bell ringing inside the room. Instead, we see two hands shaking a silver cocktail shaker through two holes cut in the door, immediately after the doorbell has been rung.[20]

The man lying on the bed in the room gives a start. The young woman goes to open the door.

Shot 171. Medium low-angle shot of a door seen from the outside. A man with a hat goes up the stairs and approaches it.

Shot 172. Camera turned 135° to the left. Close-up of the man's hand ringing a bell on the left of the frame.

Shot 173.   Close-up of two arms in white sleeves coming out of two holes in a white wall. They shake a cocktail mixer.

Shot 174.   Same as shot 170.

Shot 175.   Same as shot 173.

Shot 176.   Same as shot 174. There is an expression of restlessness on the man's face.

Shot 177.   Long medium shot of the woman crossing the room in front of the camera; she goes toward the door, opens it, and exits.

Shot 178.   Long medium low-angle shot of the man with the hat, seen from the back as he waits impatiently for someone to open the front door. The door finally opens and the man goes in. The door closes.

Shot 179.   Same as shot 176.

The stranger goes directly over to the bed and commands the man lying down to get up. The man is so reluctant to do this that the stranger is obliged to grab his cuffs and force him to rise. The newcomer tears off the man's frills one by one and hurls them out of the window along with the striped box and the thong, which the man tries vainly to save from the catastrophe. He then orders the man to go and stand against one of the walls of the room as a punishment.

Shot 180.   A door opens in front of the camera. Long shot of the man lying in bed, stretched from the right to the left of the frame. As he moves forward, the man with the hat approaches the bed. The lamp casts light on his left elbow.

Shot 181.   Medium shot of what was in the previous shot. The man with the hat signals to the man lying in bed that he wants him to get up.

Shot 182.   Dissolve to a close-up of the man lying in bed. We can see the white frills around his head and neck and the box with the striped cover. He has an expression of fear on his face.

Shot 183.   Camera turned 90° to the left. Medium shot of the headboard, the lying man's head, and the striped box. On the left of the frame we can see the plaid jacket sleeve of the man with the hat.

Shot 184.　Same as shot 182.

Shot 185.　Same as shot 183. The man with the hat bends toward the bed as he enters the frame in medium shot. He grasps the man lying in bed and shakes him about.

Shot 186.　Close-up of the man in bed as he is shaken. The box is offscreen.

Shot 187.　Camera in the same position as in shot 185. The man with the hat pulls the other man out of bed. We see the rumpled white pillow on the left of the frame.

Shot 188.　Camera turned 45° to the left. Long shot of the man with the hat, his back to the camera, as he holds the man he has just pulled out of bed. On the right of the frame we can see the window with closed curtains. The man with the hat takes away the frills the other man was wearing and moves toward the window.

Shot 189.　Medium shot of the man with the hat seen from the back. He opens the French windows and throws the frills outside.

Shot 190.　Countershot. Exterior. Long low-angle shot of the frills falling from the balcony. The balcony railing has a wrought-iron design similar to the one in shot 6, but there are no plants on the balcony. Interplay of sun and shade on the outside wall.

Shot 191.　Same as shot 189.

Shot 192.　Same as shot 190.

Shot 193.　Same as end of shot 191.

Shot 194.　Medium shot of the man with a piece of rope around his neck. He becomes aware of it and attempts to hide it in his pocket.

Shot 195.　Medium shot of the man with the hat, seen from the back, closing the French door and turning to his right.

Shot 196.　Continuation of shot 194. Caught in his attempt to hide the piece of rope, the man takes it out of his pocket and hands it to the man with the hat, who remains offscreen. We can see his hands on the right-hand side of the frame.

Shot 197.　Medium shot of the two men (the man with the hat is seen from the back as he is given the piece of rope).

Shot 198.　Medium shot of the man looking at the right of the frame.

Shot 199.   Close-up of the head of the man with the hat, seen from behind. He opens the French door and throws the piece of rope outside.

Shot 200.   Countershot. Medium low-angle shot of the balcony. The piece of rope falls on the street. Sunshine.

Shot 201.   Long medium shot of the two men. The man with the hat signals the other man to face the wall; the latter refuses to do it at first but eventually obeys the order. The camera pans on the man with the hat as he moves to the left-hand side of the frame and disappears; the other man stands facing the wall next to the tennis racket, holding his hands in a childish pose (see shot 125).

Shot 202.   Medium shot of the man facing the wall. His head touches the wall right next to the tennis racket. He turns to the camera, then resumes his position.

Shot 203.   Medium shot of the man with his head against the wall. In the foreground, the man with the hat, seen from behind, signals him to pull up his arms.

Shot 204.   Medium shot of the man facing the wall with his arms crossed.

Shot 205.   Same as end of shot 203.

Shot 206.   Same as shot 204.

Shot 207.   Long medium shot of the man with the hat hiding almost entirely the other man's body. He takes off his hat, casts it to his right, and begins to turn. At this moment the tango music stops and Wagner music starts playing again.

On a black screen the following words appear:

Seize ans avant. (Sixteen years before.)

The stranger has done all this with his back to the camera. Only now does he turn around for the first time to go and fetch something in another part of the room. At that instant, the shot goes out of focus. The stranger moves in slow motion and we see that his features are identical to those of the first man. They are the same person, except that the stranger is younger, more full of pathos, rather like the man must have been many years earlier.

Shot 208.   The man who wore the hat (now without the hat, man no. 2) turns in slow motion. He has the same face as the man against the wall. He moves toward the camera, wringing his hands in distress. He wears a gray necktie with black and white diagonal stripes around his tuxedo collar.

The stranger walks across the room, while the camera tracks back to reveal him in medium close-up. He is walking toward an old school desk that now comes into shot. There are various school things lying about on the desk, including two books. The placing of the objects must have a clear and symbolic meaning.[21]

The stranger picks up the books and turns to go back toward the man. In that instant, the shot ceases to be out of focus and in slow motion, and goes back to normal.

Shot 209.   Close-up of a school desk placed diagonally in the frame, from the lower left to the upper right. There is a notebook in the upper left side, a chalk eraser in the upper right corner, an open book in the foreground, and a quill in an inkwell.

Shot 210.   Long medium shot of man no. 2 approaching the school desk. The objects described in the previous shot have a different position, thus breaking the *raccord* of the point of view. In the background, on the left, man no. 1 is still facing the wall.

Shot 211.   Same as shot 209. The hands of man no. 2 enter the frame from the lower left, close the book and notebook, and take them away.

Shot 212.   Same as shot 210. Man no. 2 turns to man no. 1 with the book and the notebook in his hands.

Shot 213.   At this point a perfect *raccord* of movement ends the slow motion, while keeping the same camera position and the same elements in the frame. Man no. 2 moves toward man no. 1.

When the stranger reaches the spot where the other man is standing, he orders him to stretch out his arms in the shape of a cross and places a book in each of the man's hands, ordering him to keep this position as a punishment.

Shot 214.   Same as shot 204. Man no. 1 looks to the right of the frame.

Shot 215.   Medium shot of the two men facing each other, separated by the door crossbar.[22] Man no. 1 is on the right-hand side of the frame, man no. 2 on the left.

Shot 216.   Medium shot of man no. 1 with his arms stretched to the right of the frame. Two hands, each holding one book, appear in the lower right. Man no. 1 takes them and crosses his arms again with a strange smile on his face.

Shot 217.   Close-up of man no. 2 in the middle part of the frame as he moves his head in slow motion with an expression of pain on his face.

The man looks vicious and treacherous as he turns to face the stranger. The books he is holding begin to change into two revolvers. The stranger looks at the man with an expression of ever-increasing tenderness. The man threatens the stranger with his guns, forcing him to put his hands up. In spite of this, the first man fires both revolvers.

Shot 218.   Medium shot of man no. 2 standing sideways to the camera as he moves in the direction of man no. 1. We see only the latter's right arm holding a book in an oblique position. Man no. 2 turns and moves in the direction of the camera. End of slow motion.

Shot 219.   Long medium shot of man no. 1 turning to the right as he holds the books.

Shot 220.   Medium shot of man no. 2, seen from the back as he moves away toward a door. On the right-hand side of the frame is a mirror, where we see the man's reflection. When the image disappears from the mirror, cut to

Shot 221.   Same as shot 219. Suddenly the two books become guns aimed at man no. 2 as man no. 1 signals man no. 2 to put his hands up.

Shot 222.   Long medium shot of man no. 2 reaching the door; he stops and then turns to man no. 1.

Shot 223.   Close-up of the head of man no. 2 seen from the back. He has a different hairstyle. When he moves to the right, man no. 1 appears on the left of the frame in the background. He also has a different hairstyle and aims the two guns at the other man.

Shot 224.   Camera turned 45° to the left. Long medium shot of man no. 1 aiming his guns.

Shot 225.   Same as end of shot 223.

Shot 226.   Close-up of man no. 2 with his hands up. Slow motion.

Shot 227.   Medium shot of man no. 1 with the gun in his left hand, signaling man no. 2 (offscreen) to put up his hands. Return to natural motion.

Shot 228.   Same as shot 226. Slow motion.

Shot 229.   Same as shot 227. Man no. 1 begins shooting with a sadistic expression. Return to natural motion.

Shot 230.   Same as shot 225. Man no. 2 begins to fall.

Shot 231.   Same as shot 228. Man no. 2 begins a back fall. Slow motion.

Shot 232.   Camera turned 45° compared to shot 227. Close-up of the guns shooting. Return to natural motion.

Medium close-up of the stranger falling to the ground, mortally wounded, an expression of pain contorting his features (the photography is once again out of focus and in even slower motion).

In the distance, we see the wounded man, no longer inside the room, but in a park. By him sits a woman with bare shoulders, her back turned to the camera, leaning slightly forward.

As he falls, the wounded man tries to grasp and stroke the woman's bare shoulders; one of his trembling hands is turned inward, while the other lightly claws at the bare skin. The man finally falls to the ground.

Shot 233.   Same as shot 231. Man no. 2 falls backward, a blank expression on his face. Slow motion.

Shot 234.   Man no. 2 falls forward. Low-angle close-up. We are no longer in a room, but outside. Behind the man's head as he falls we can see leaves from a tree. Return to natural motion.

Shot 235.   Long shot of man no. 2 as he falls over the naked torso of a woman seated in a meadow and slightly bent forward. A creek flows in the background.

Shot 236.   Close-up of a woman's naked torso. She wears the same neck-lace and earrings as the woman at the beginning of the film. As he falls, the man tries to hold on to her naked shoulder, the palm of his left hand turned to the camera, his right hand attempting to grab her shoulder; his hands slide for lack of strength, and disappear from the frame.

Shot 237.   Same as shot 235. The woman is gone; only the man's body lies on the grass.

Long shot: a few passers-by and a policeman rush over to the man, pick him up, and carry him off through the woods. Let the passionate lame man take part.[23]

Shot 238.   Long shot of the meadow. The man's body lies in the middle. Four men wearing hats enter the frame from the four corners and approach the man.

Shot 239.   Long shot of two men. The one not wearing a hat, his hair combed back, wears a gray necktie with black and white di-agonal stripes, a handkerchief in the upper pocket of his jacket, and his hands are in the pockets of his pants. The one accom-panying him wears a hat and a plain necktie, and has a stick. The two men move in the meadow in the direction of the camera.

Shot 240.   Close-up of the four men walking around the body lying on the grass. One of them seems to be looking for something in his in-side jacket pocket; someone interrupts him. Another suggests sending for help and bends to listen to the lying man's heartbeat.

Shot 241.   Continuation of shot 239.

Shot 242.   Same as shot 240.

Shot 243.   Long shot of the two men from shot 241 crossing the frame from left to right. The camera tracks them. The man that left the group in shot 240 enters from the left and joins them.

Shot 244.   Camera turned. Medium shot of the three men speaking.

Shot 245.   Camera turned again. The men split up. The two men from shot 241 disappear from the lower right of the frame, the third man through the lower left.

Shot 246.   Same as shot 237 in long shot. The third man enters the frame running from the left of the frame. The two men from shot 241 do the same a little later, abruptly breaking the *raccord* with the previous shot. The man without the hat, who does not even look at the fallen body, seems to tell the others to pick up the body and take it away. He turns his back to the group as they do this and then walks after them.

Shot 247.   Long shot of the men carrying the body. The man with the stick leads them. The man without the hat follows the three men at a distance. They move toward the camera.

Shot 248.   Close-up of the group, shot from the same position with a hand-held camera.

Shot 249.   Same as shot 247.

Shot 250.   Dissolve with the camera turned 180° to a long high-angle shot of the four men moving away from the camera. Fade-out. The tango music starts again in the sound track.

Cut back to the same room. The door in which the man's hand was caught now opens slowly. The young woman appears. She closes the door behind her and carefully examines the wall against which the murderer was just standing.

The man is no longer there. The wall is blank; there is no furniture or decoration on it.[24] *The young woman makes a gesture of annoyance and impatience.*

Shot 251.   Fade-in to a close-up of a door. On the right of the frame, the same piece of furniture (lacquer) with the mirror as in shot 220. The door opens and the woman appears. Tango no. 1 starts again.

Shot 252.   Dissolve to a medium shot of the woman closing the door behind her and then leaning against it with a pensive expression and a blank gaze.

Shot of the wall again. There is a small black spot in the middle of it. This little spot, seen closer in, is a death's-head moth. Close-up of the moth, large close-up of the death's-head on its back. The death's-head covers the whole screen.[25]

Shot 253.   Long shot of a moth on white background in the lower part of the frame, placed diagonally from the lower right to the upper left of the screen.

Shot 254.   Dissolve to a medium long shot of the moth.

Shot 255.   Same as shot 252.

Shot 256.   Same as shot 254.

Shot 257.   Dissolve to a close-up of the moth placed diagonally but in the opposite sense. Iris-out to a death's-head inscribed on its back between the wings.

Shot 258.   Close-up of the death's-head.

Shot 259.   Close-up of a woman's face in the middle of the frame looking with displeasure to the offscreen space on the right-hand side of the camera.

Shot 260.   Same as shot 258.

Medium close-up of the man who was wearing the frills. He suddenly claps his hand to his mouth as though his teeth were falling out. The young woman looks at him disdainfully. When the man takes his hand away, we see his mouth has disappeared.

Shot 261.   Camera turned from its position in shot 259. Medium shot of man no. 1 looking at the offscreen space on the right-hand side of the camera. He wears a dark, double-breasted suit and a necktie with diagonal black and white stripes (see shot 43); his hair is combed back.

Shot 262.   Camera turned. Medium shot of the previous shot.

Shot 263.   Camera turned. Same as shot 261. The man suddenly claps his right hand to his mouth.

Shot 264.   Camera turned. Same as shot 259, an expression of displeasure on the woman's face.

Shot 265.   Camera turned. Same as shot 263. When the man takes his hand down, his mouth has disappeared.

The young woman seems to say to him, "Well, and afterward?" Then she redoes her lips with her lipstick.

Shot 266.   Camera turned. Same as shot 262. The woman takes a lipstick out of her purse and frantically applies lipstick to her lips.

On the man's face, hairs are growing in the place where his mouth used to be. When the young woman notices, she stifles a cry and quickly looks at her armpit which is completely hairless.[26]

Shot 267.   Medium shot of the man; the hair of an armpit has been superimposed on his mouth.

Shot 268.   Same as shot 262. The woman drops the lipstick and looks with astonishment at her hairless armpit.

Shot 269.   Close-up of the armpit.

Shot 270.   Long shot of the woman with the camera placed behind the man's head. In the middle of the frame is the piece of furniture with the mirror (see shots 220 and 251).

Shot 271.   Long medium shot of the woman, who picks up a handkerchief, wraps it around her neck, and makes a move to open the door.

Shot 272.   Same as end of shot 267.

She scornfully thrusts out her tongue at the man, throws a shawl over her shoulders, and opens the door. She walks out of the door into the next room, which is a vast beach.[27]

Shot 273.   Close-up of the woman sticking her tongue out to the man as she stands by the door. She exits and closes the door.

Shot 274.   Same as shot 270, with the woman gone. The door is slightly open.

Shot 275.   Same as shot 273, with the camera moved slightly forward. The woman's tongue remains offscreen.

Shot 276.   Camera turned 90° to the right. Medium shot of the woman sticking out her tongue as she leans into the room from the door.

She closes the door and turns. The wind moves the handkerchief —which has vertical black stripes on a white background— around her neck and forces her to half-close her eyes.

A man is waiting by the edge of the sea. This man and the young woman seem happy to see each other; they wander off together down the beach, following the shoreline.[28]

Shot 277.   Long shot of a man with his arms akimbo looking at the sea from a stony beach. He wears a sweater with horizontal stripes. A little boat sails in the distance. The man turns and moves toward the camera.

Shot 278.   Same as end of shot 276. The woman waves warmly at the man as she moves forward. She disappears from the frame.

Shot 279.   Camera turned. Long medium shot of the man with the striped sweater, his arms akimbo, looking to the right of the frame. He wears a gray necktie with black and white diagonal stripes.

Shot 280.   Long shot of the beach. The man is on the left of the frame. The woman, with her back to the camera, moves toward the man with a loving expression.

Shot 281.   Medium shot of the man and the woman. She seems to speak in an affectionate manner. He turns his head to the other side and, by way of reply, shows her his wristwatch, as though to indicate displeasure for her delay.

Shot 282.   Camera turned 180°. Close-up of the woman looking at the man's watch on the right-hand side of the frame. In the background we can briefly see the rectangular railings of the beach embankment.

Shot 283.   Camera turned 180°. Medium shot of the woman caressing and embracing the man. He persists in his annoyed attitude, keeping his head turned to the other side. She holds his face and kisses him. Finally he responds to her fondling and kisses her.

Shot of their legs and the waves at their feet.

Camera tracks after the couple. The waves gently wash up the thong, the striped box, the frills, and, last of all, the bicycle. Camera remains fixed for a while, even though nothing more is being washed ashore.[29]

Shot 284.   Dissolve to a long shot of the man and the woman with their backs to the camera as they walk away on the beach with their arms around each other's waists.

Shot 285.   Camera turned 135° to the left. Long shot of the man and the woman seen from the front as they walk along the beach in the same attitude as in the previous shot. They walk with difficulty on the rocks. The waves break softly on the sand.

Shot 286.   Medium medium high-angle shot of a broken box on the beach rocks. The man and the woman (we can see only their legs from the knees down) enter the frame from the left.

Shot 287.   Close-up of the broken box. The cover has diagonal black and white stripes. There are also dirty white frills and a piece of rope. The man kicks the box.

The two people wander down the beach, gradually fading from view as the following words appear in the sky:

Shot 288.   Same as shot 286, without the box. The woman bends, picks up the frills and the rope, and hands them to the man, who hurls them aside with a spiteful gesture. They hold each other from the waist again, resume walking, and disappear from the left-hand side of the frame.

Shot 289.   Dissolve to a shot that is identical to shot 283. Toward the end the following words appear:

Au printemps . . . (In spring . . .)

Everything has changed. We now see a limitless desert; the man and the young woman are in the center of the screen, buried up to their chests in sand, blinded, in rags, being eaten alive by the sun and by swarms of insects.[30]

Fade out to a black screen where the same words appear.

Shot 290.   Fade-in (the words are kept in superimposition for half of the shot) to the two people on the beach sunk in the sand up to their chests, in an aesthetic attitude. On the left, a woman with her head turned to the sky; on the right, a man with his head turned to the ground. Behind his back we can see two cross-shaped wooden bars supporting him as a sort of scaffolding. There are dunes and a gray sky behind them. Fade to black. On a rough background appears the word

FIN (THE END)

Fade to black.

Appendix 2
Découpage of *Un Chien andalou*

The photographic découpage that follows is based on the standard Spanish copy of the film. Differences between cuts or fades and dissolves are maintained. The dissolves are indicated by including one photogram from the shot immediately preceding the dissolve, one photogram from the superimposition, and one photogram from the new shot. Numerically, the dissolves are considered autonomous shots, with the exception only of shot 48. In this case, the dissolve that transforms the unbuttoned collar and loose necktie into a buttoned collar with a knotted necktie results from editing within the shot (as part of the mise-en-scène) and not from editing in the sequence (territory of the temporal discursive linearity) aimed at producing a visual rhyme effect with shot 46; consequently, shot 48 does not constitute a shot in itself. Credits and intertitles are not included in the numbering of the shots.

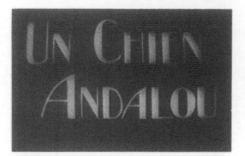

Photogram 1

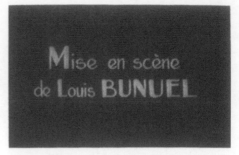

Photogram 2

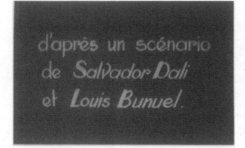

Photogram 3

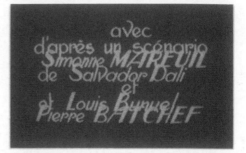

Photogram 4

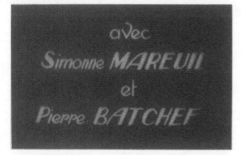

Photogram 5

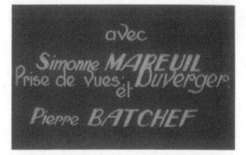

Photogram 6

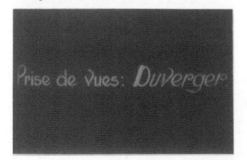

Photogram 7

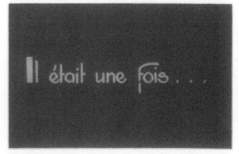

Photogram 8

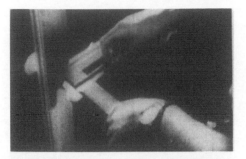

Photogram 9/Shot 1

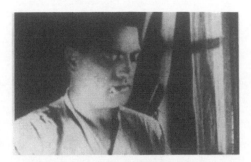

Photogram 10/Shot 2

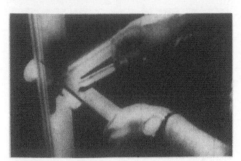

Photogram 11/Shot 3a

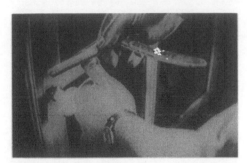

Photogram 12/Shot 3b

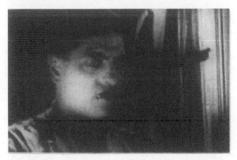

Photogram 13/Shot 4

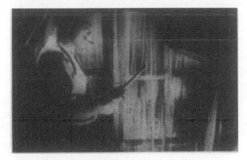

Photogram 14/Shot 5a

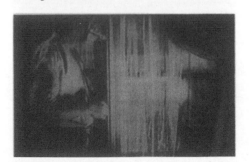

Photogram 15/Shot 5b

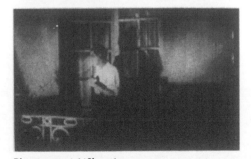

Photogram 16/Shot 6a

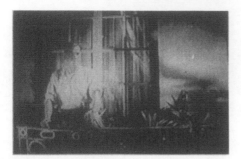

Photogram 17/Shot 6b

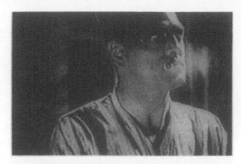

Photogram 18/Shot 7

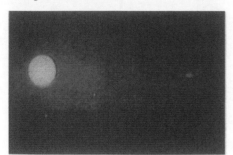

Photogram 19/Shot 8

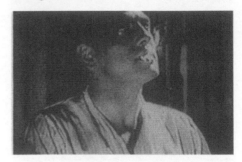

Photogram 20/Shot 9

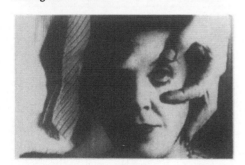

Photogram 21/Shot 10a

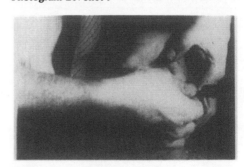

Photogram 22/Shot 10b

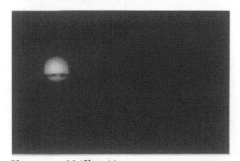

Photogram 23/Shot 11

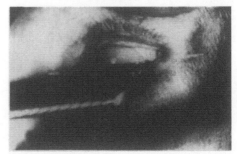

Photogram 24/Shot 12

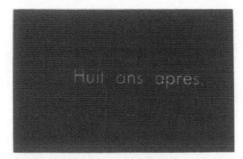

Photogram 25

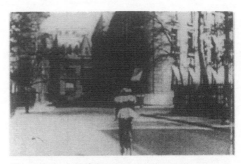

Photogram 26/Shot 13

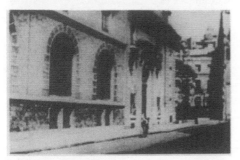

Photogram 27/Shot 14

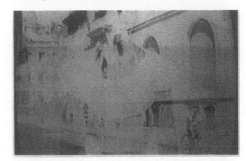

Photogram 28/Shot 15a

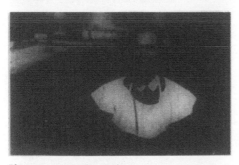

Photogram 29/Shot 15b

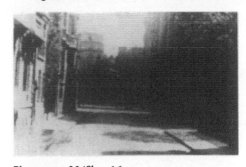

Photogram 30/Shot 16

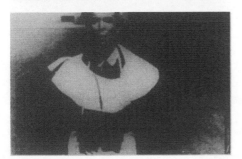

Photogram 31/Shot 17

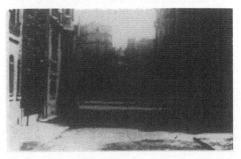

Photogram 32/Shot 18

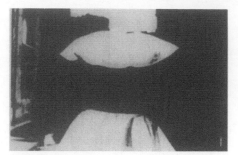

Photogram 33 / Shot 19a

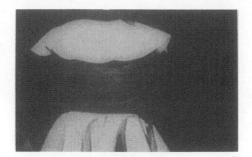

Photogram 34 / Shot 19b

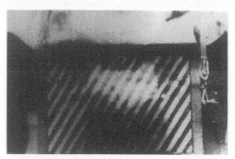

Photogram 35 / Shot 19c

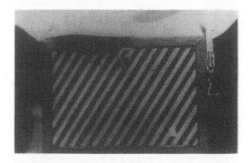

Photogram 36 / Shot 20

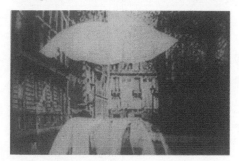

Photogram 37 / Shot 21a

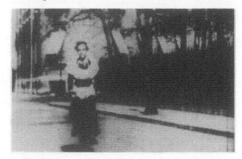

Photogram 38 / Shot 21b

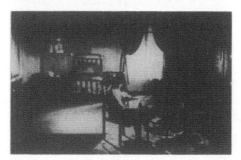

Photogram 39 / Shot 22

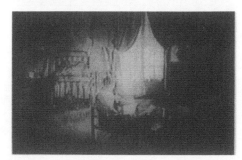

Photogram 40 / Shot 23a

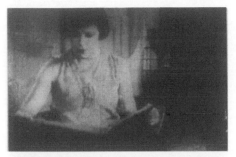

Photogram 41/Shot 23b

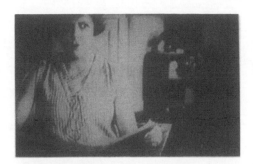

Photogram 42/Shot 23c

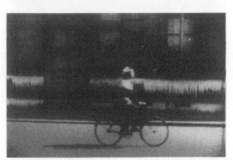

Photogram 43/Shot 24

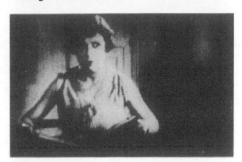

Photogram 44/Shot 25

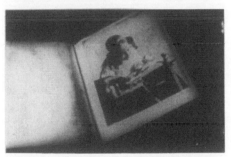

Photogram 45/Shot 26

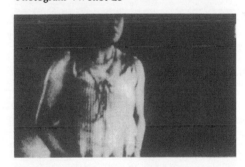

Photogram 46/Shot 27

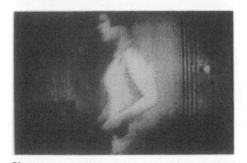

Photogram 47/Shot 28a

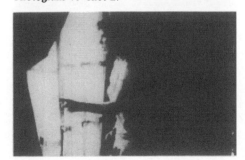

Photogram 48/Shot 28b

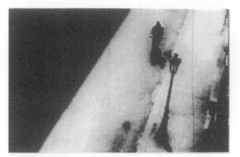

Photogram 49/Shot 29

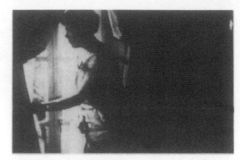

Photogram 50/Shot 30

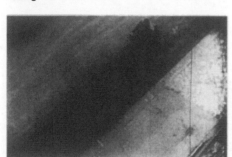

Photogram 51/Shot 31a

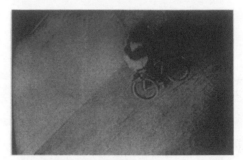

Photogram 52/Shot 31b

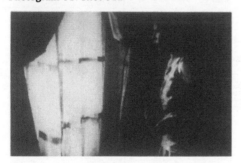

Photogram 53/Shot 32

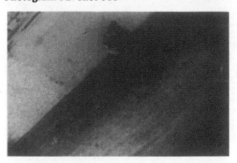

Photogram 54/Shot 33

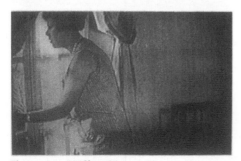

Photogram 55/Shot 34

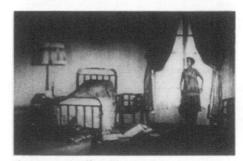

Photogram 56/Shot 35

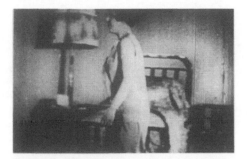

Photogram 57/Shot 36a

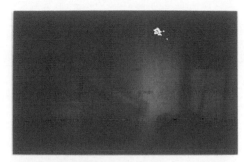

Photogram 58/Shot 36b

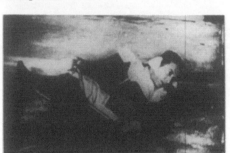

Photogram 59/Shot 37

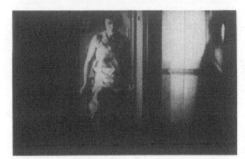

Photogram 60/Shot 38

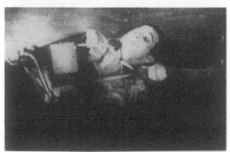

Photogram 61/Shot 39

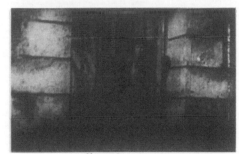

Photogram 62/Shot 40

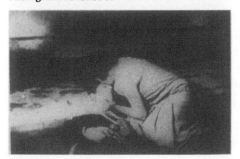

Photogram 63/Shot 41

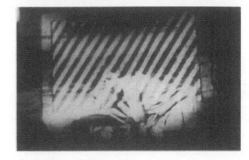

Photogram 64/Shot 42a

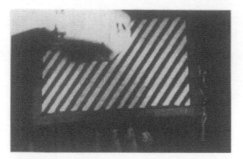

Photogram 65/Shot 42b

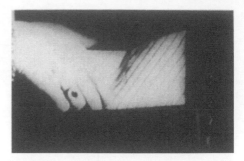

Photogram 66/Shot 42c

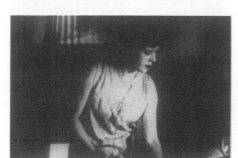

Photogram 67/Shot 43a

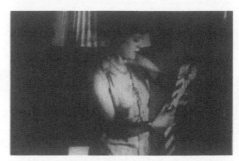

Photogram 68/Shot 43b

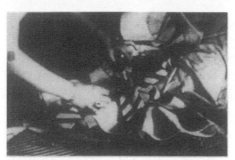

Photogram 69/Shot 44

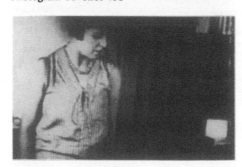

Photogram 70/Shot 45a

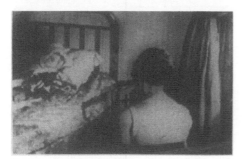

Photogram 71/Shot 45b

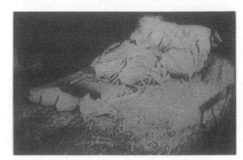

Photogram 72/Shot 46a

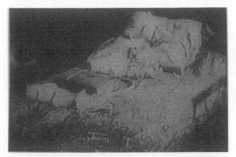

Photogram 73/Shot 46b

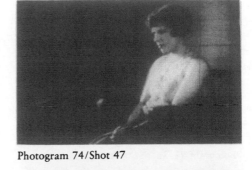

Photogram 74/Shot 47

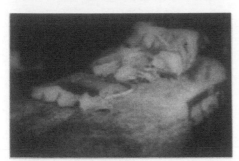

Photogram 75/Shot 48a

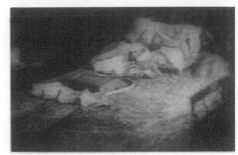

Photogram 76/Shot 48b

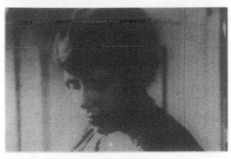

Photogram 77/Shot 49a

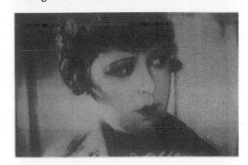

Photogram 78/Shot 49b

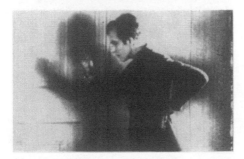

Photogram 79/Shot 50

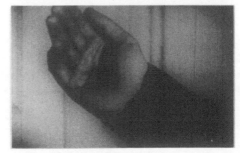

Photogram 80/Shot 51

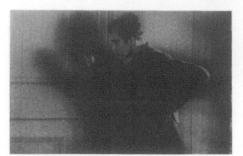

Photogram 81/Shot 52

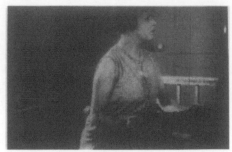

Photogram 82/Shot 53

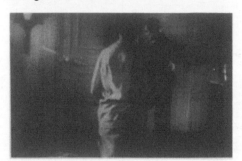

Photogram 83/Shot 54

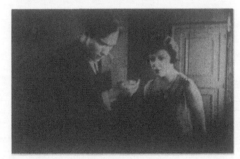

Photogram 84/Shot 55

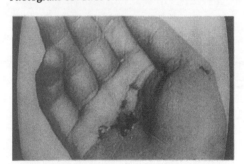

Photogram 85/Shot 56

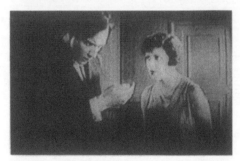

Photogram 86/Shot 57a

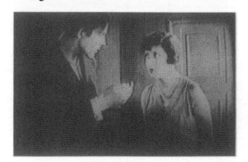

Photogram 87/Shot 57b

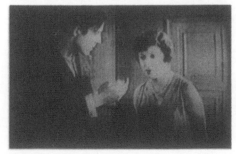

Photogram 88/Shot 57c

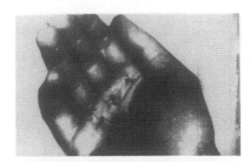

Photogram 89/Shot 57d

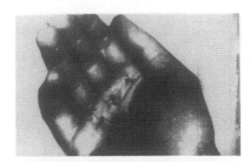

Photogram 90/Shot 58

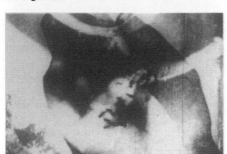

Photogram 91/Shot 59a

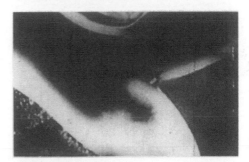

Photogram 92/Shot 59b

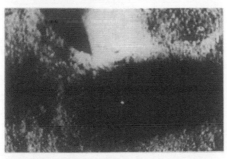

Photogram 93/Shot 60a

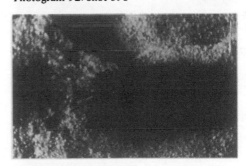

Photogram 94/Shot 60b

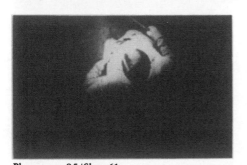

Photogram 95/Shot 61

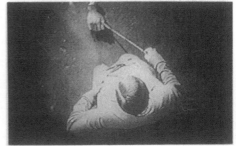

Photogram 96/Shot 62

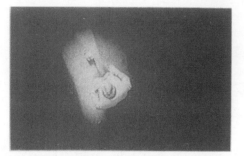

Photogram 97/Shot 63a

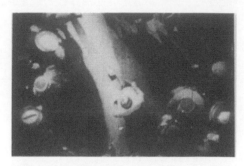

Photogram 98/Shot 63b

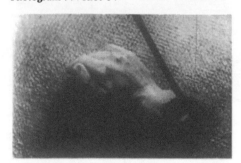

Photogram 99/Shot 64

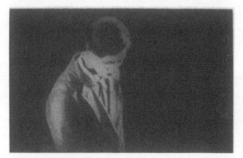

Photogram 100/Shot 65

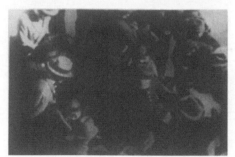

Photogram 101/Shot 66

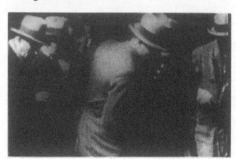

Photogram 102/Shot 67

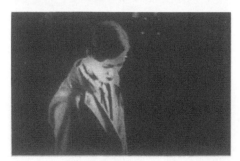

Photogram 103/Shot 68

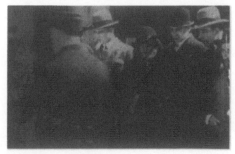

Photogram 104/Shot 69

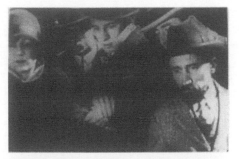

Photogram 105/Shot 70

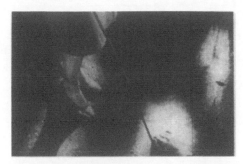

Photogram 106/Shot 71

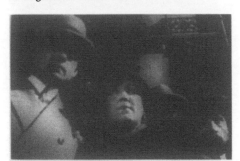

Photogram 107/Shot 72

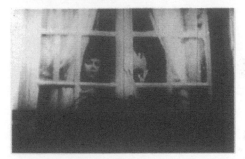

Photogram 108/Shot 73

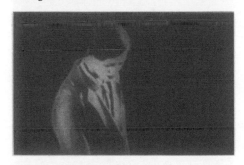

Photogram 109/Shot 74

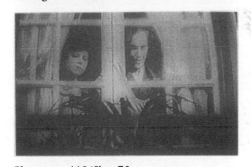

Photogram 110/Shot 75

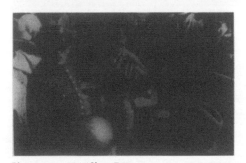

Photogram 111/Shot 76

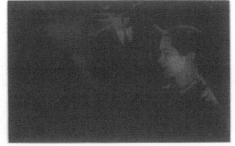

Photogram 112/Shot 77

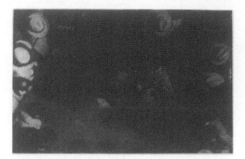

Photogram 113/Shot 78

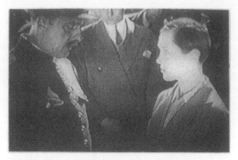

Photogram 114/Shot 79

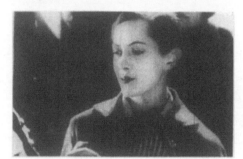

Photogram 115/Shot 80

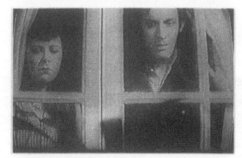

Photogram 116/Shot 81a

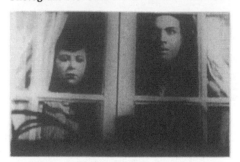

Photogram 117/Shot 81b

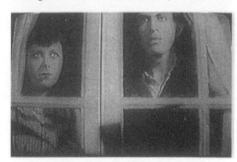

Photogram 118/Shot 81c

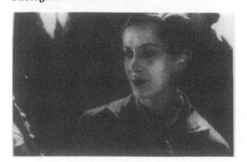

Photogram 119/Shot 82

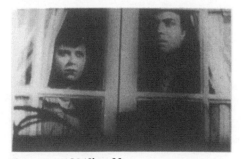

Photogram 120/Shot 83

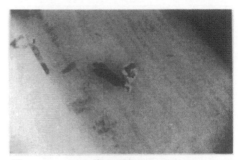

Photogram 121/Shot 84a

Photogram 122/Shot 84b

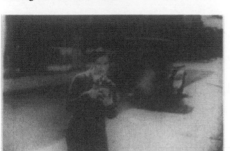

Photogram 123/Shot 85

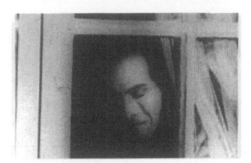

Photogram 124/Shot 86

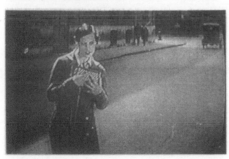

Photogram 125/Shot 87

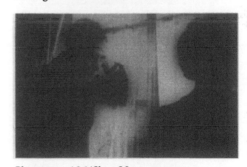

Photogram 126/Shot 88

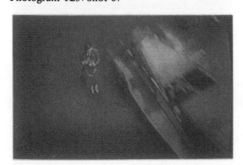

Photogram 127/Shot 89

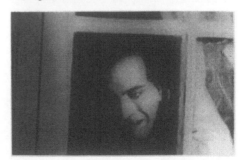

Photogram 128/Shot 90

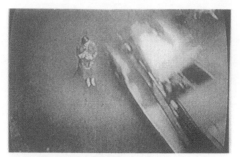

Photogram 129/Shot 91

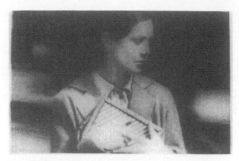

Photogram 130/Shot 92

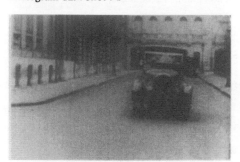

Photogram 131/Shot 93

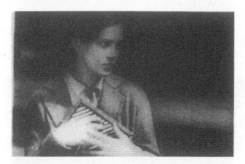

Photogram 132/Shot 94

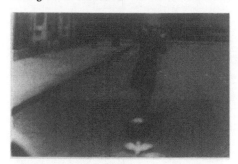

Photogram 133/Shot 95

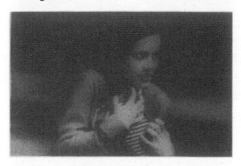

Photogram 134/Shot 96

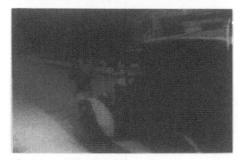

Photogram 135/Shot 97

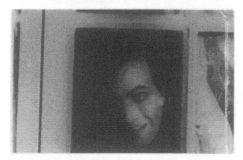

Photogram 136/Shot 98

Photogram 137/Shot 99a

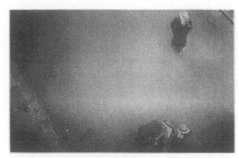

Photogram 138/Shot 99b

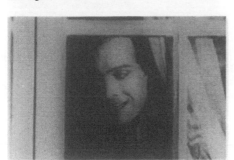

Photogram 139/Shot 100a

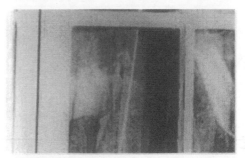

Photogram 140/Shot 100b

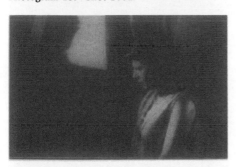

Photogram 141/Shot 101

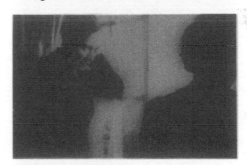

Photogram 142/Shot 102

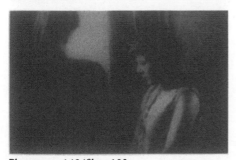

Photogram 143/Shot 103

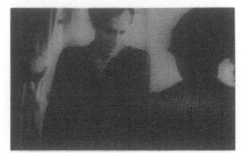

Photogram 144/Shot 104

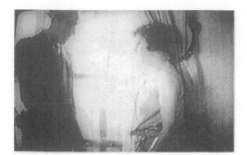

Photogram 145/Shot 105a

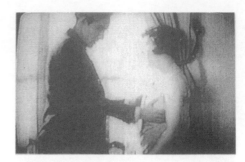

Photogram 146/Shot 105b

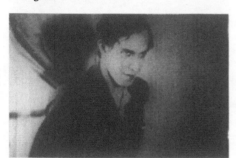

Photogram 147/Shot 106

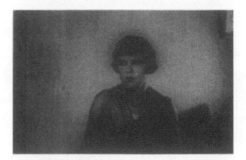

Photogram 148/Shot 107

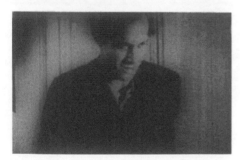

Photogram 149/Shot 108

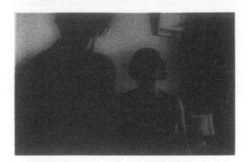

Photogram 150/Shot 109a

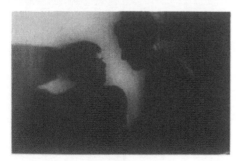

Photogram 151/Shot 109b

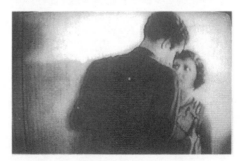

Photogram 152/Shot 109c

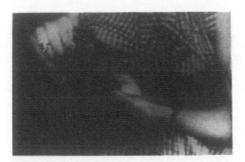

Photogram 153/Shot 110

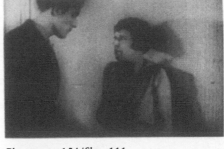

Photogram 154/Shot 111

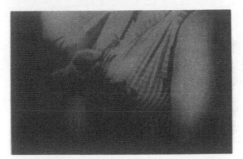

Photogram 155/Shot 112

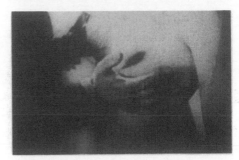

Photogram 156/Shot 113a

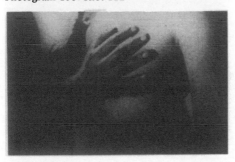

Photogram 157/Shot 113b

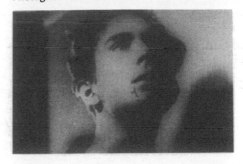

Photogram 158/Shot 114

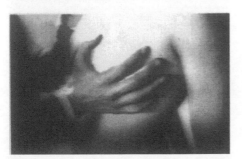

Photogram 159/Shot 115

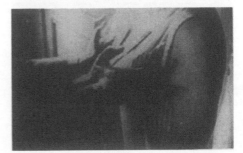

Photogram 160/Shot 116

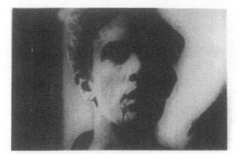

Photogram 161/Shot 117

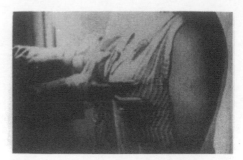

Photogram 162/Shot 118

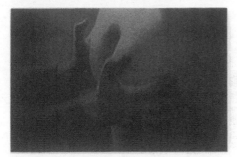

Photogram 163/Shot 119

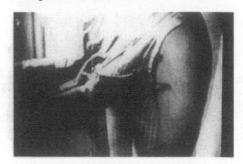

Photogram 164/Shot 120

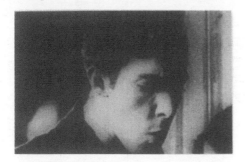

Photogram 165/Shot 121

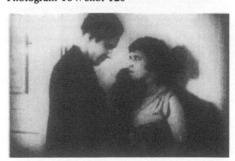

Photogram 166/Shot 122

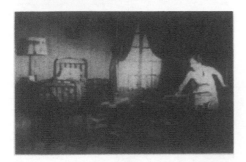

Photogram 167/Shot 123a

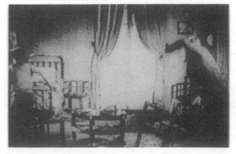

Photogram 168/Shot 123b

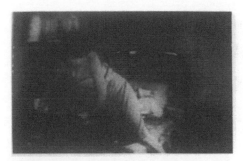

Photogram 169/Shot 124a

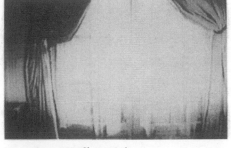

Photogram 170/Shot 124b

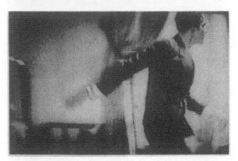

Photogram 171/Shot 124c

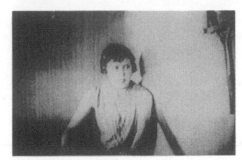

Photogram 172/Shot 125a

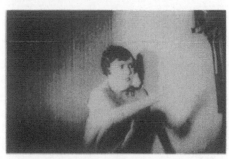

Photogram 173/Shot 125b

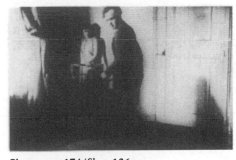

Photogram 174/Shot 126

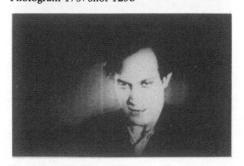

Photogram 175/Shot 127

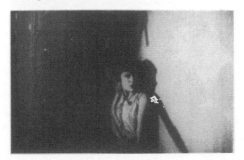

Photogram 176/Shot 128

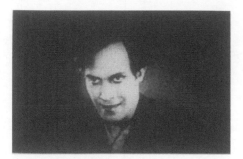

Photogram 177/Shot 129

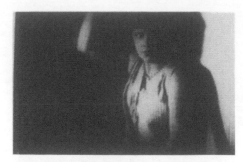

Photogram 178/Shot 130

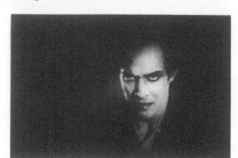

Photogram 179/Shot 131

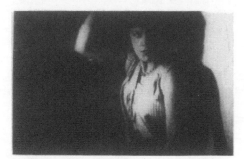

Photogram 180/Shot 132

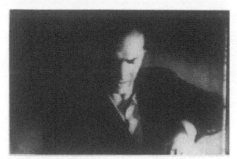

Photogram 181/Shot 133

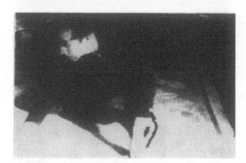

Photogram 182/Shot 134

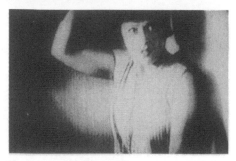

Photogram 183/Shot 135

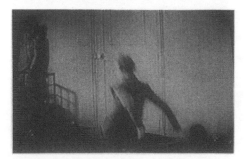

Photogram 184/Shot 136a

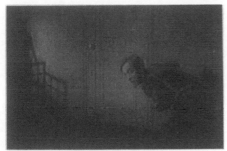

Photogram 185/Shot 136b

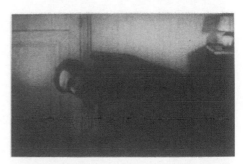

Photogram 186/Shot 137

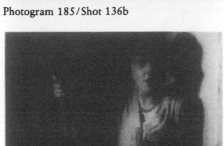

Photogram 187/Shot 138

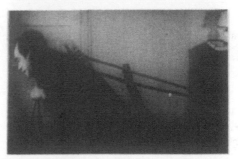

Photogram 188/Shot 139

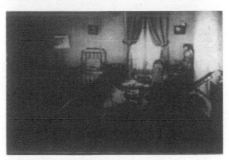

Photogram 189/Shot 140

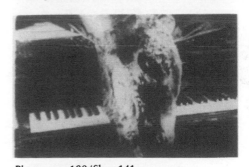

Photogram 190/Shot 141

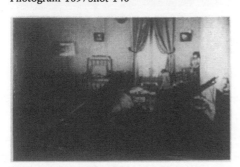

Photogram 191/Shot 142

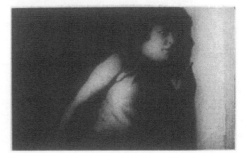

Photogram 192/Shot 143

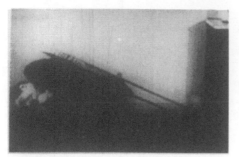

Photogram 193/Shot 144

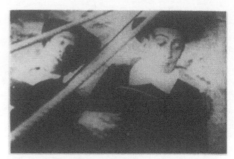

Photogram 194/Shot 145

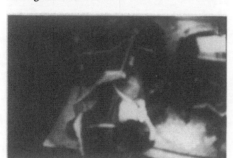

Photogram 195/Shot 146

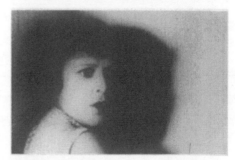

Photogram 196/Shot 147

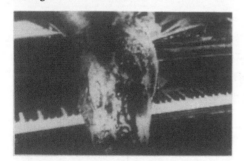

Photogram 197/Shot 148

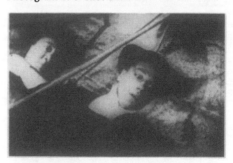

Photogram 198/Shot 149

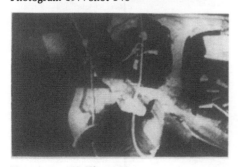

Photogram 199/Shot 150

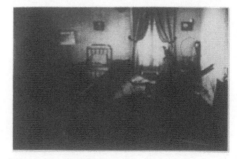

Photogram 200/Shot 151

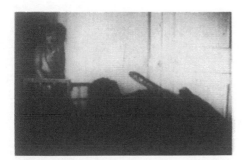

Photogram 201/Shot 152

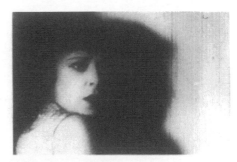

Photogram 202/Shot 153

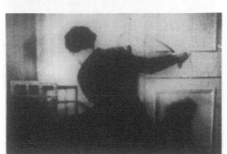

Photogram 203/Shot 154

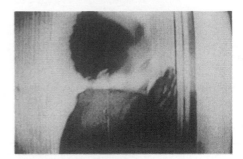

Photogram 204/Shot 155

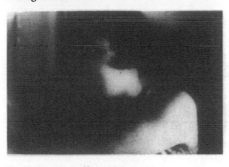

Photogram 205/Shot 156

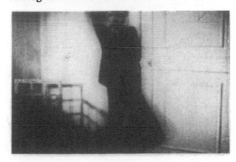

Photogram 206/Shot 157

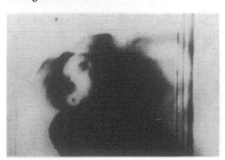

Photogram 207/Shot 158

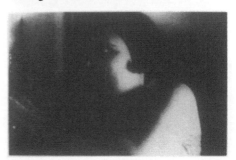

Photogram 208/Shot 159

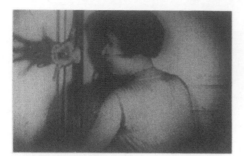

Photogram 209/Shot 160

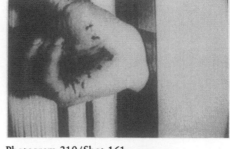

Photogram 210/Shot 161

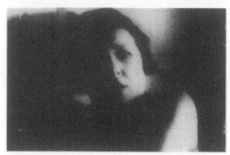

Photogram 211/Shot 162

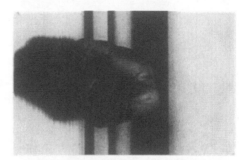

Photogram 212/Shot 163

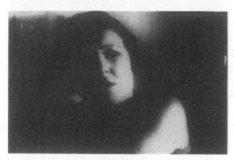

Photogram 213/Shot 164

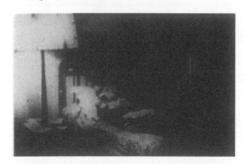

Photogram 214/Shot 165

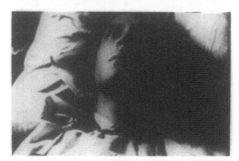

Photogram 215/Shot 166

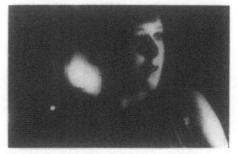

Photogram 216/Shot 167

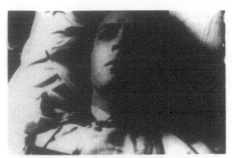

Photogram 217/Shot 168

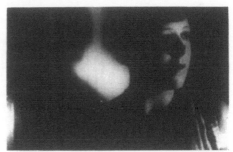

Photogram 218/Shot 169

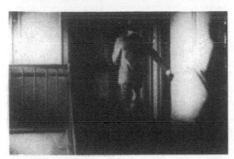

Photogram 219/Shot 170

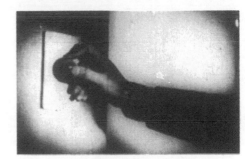

Vers trois heures du matin

Photogram 220

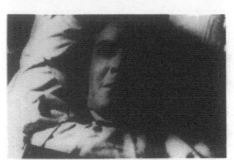

Photogram 221/Shot 171

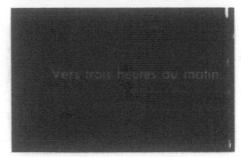

Photogram 222/Shot 172

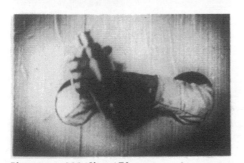

Photogram 223/Shot 173

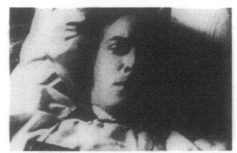

Photogram 224/Shot 174

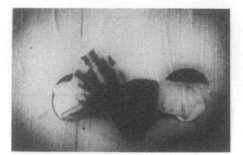

Photogram 225/Shot 175

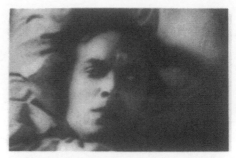

Photogram 226/Shot 176

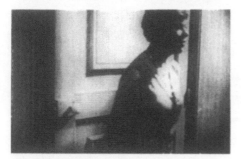

Photogram 227/Shot 177a

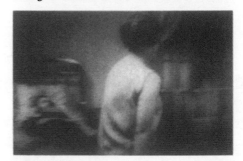

Photogram 228/Shot 177b

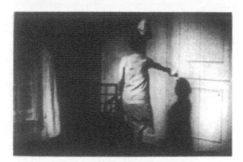

Photogram 229/Shot 177c

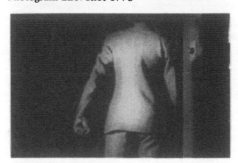

Photogram 230/Shot 178

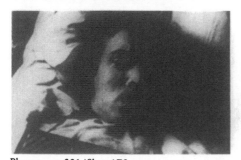

Photogram 231/Shot 179

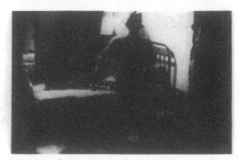

Photogram 232/Shot 180

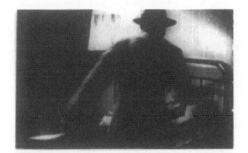

Photogram 233/Shot 181

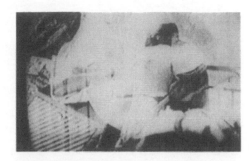

Photogram 234/Shot 182a

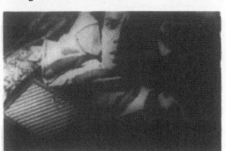

Photogram 235/Shot 182b

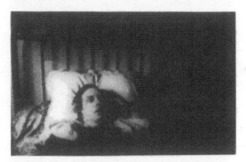

Photogram 236/Shot 183

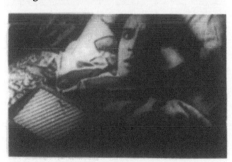

Photogram 237/Shot 184

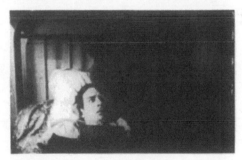

Photogram 238/Shot 185

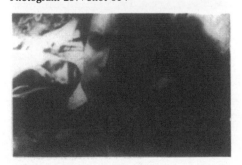

Photogram 239/Shot 186

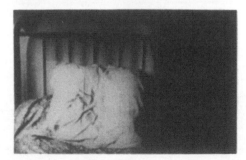

Photogram 240/Shot 187

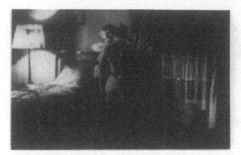

Photogram 241/Shot 188a

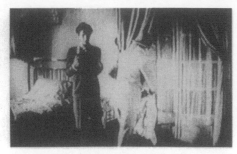

Photogram 242/Shot 188b

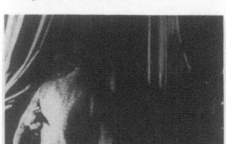

Photogram 243/Shot 189

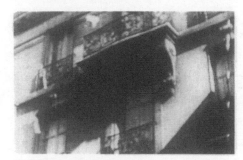

Photogram 244/Shot 190

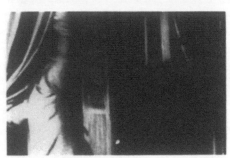

Photogram 245/Shot 191

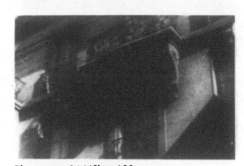

Photogram 246/Shot 192

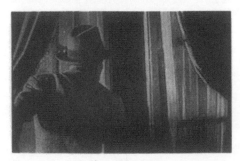

Photogram 247/Shot 193

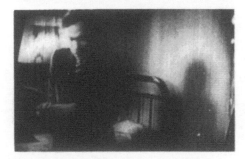

Photogram 248/Shot 194

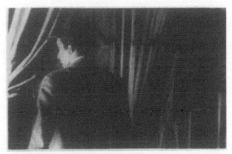

Photogram 249/Shot 195

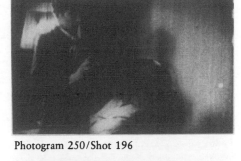

Photogram 250/Shot 196

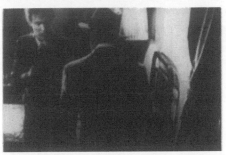

Photogram 251/Shot 197

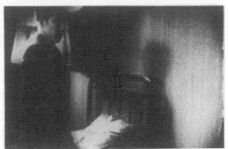

Photogram 252/Shot 198

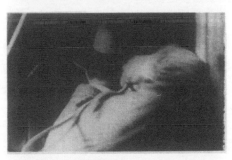

Photogram 253/Shot 199

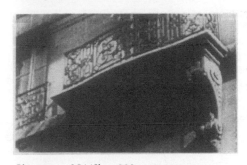

Photogram 254/Shot 200

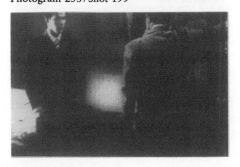

Photogram 255/Shot 201

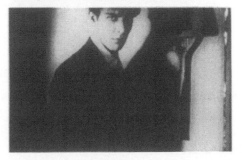

Photogram 256/Shot 202

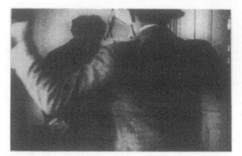

Photogram 257/Shot 203

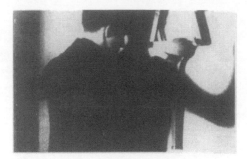

Photogram 258/Shot 204

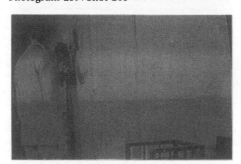

Photogram 259/Shot 205

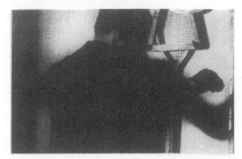

Photogram 260/Shot 206

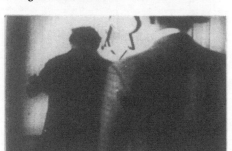

Photogram 261/Shot 207

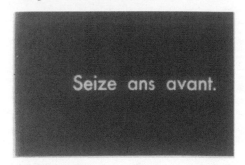

Seize ans avant.

Photogram 262

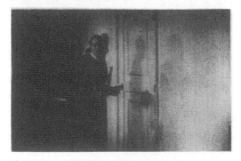

Photogram 263/Shot 208a

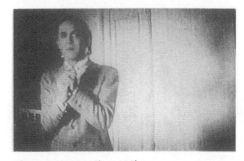

Photogram 264/Shot 208b

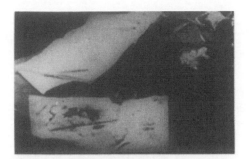

Photogram 265/Shot 209

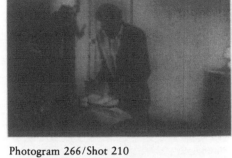

Photogram 266/Shot 210

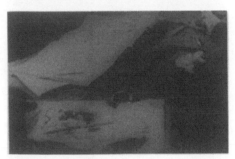

Photogram 267/Shot 211

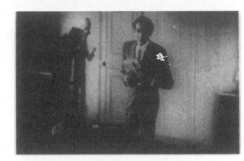

Photogram 268/Shot 212

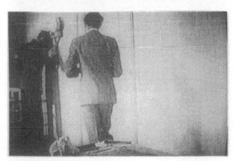

Photogram 269/Shot 213

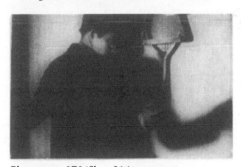

Photogram 270/Shot 214

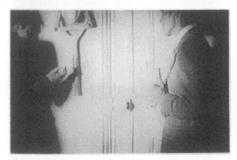

Photogram 271/Shot 215

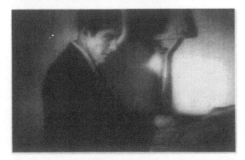

Photogram 272/Shot 216

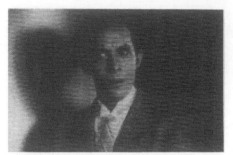

Photogram 273/Shot 217

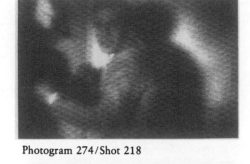

Photogram 274/Shot 218

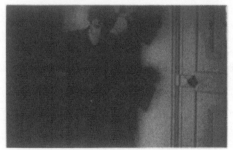

Photogram 275/Shot 219

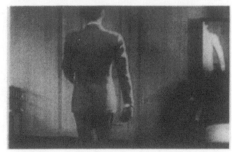

Photogram 276/Shot 220

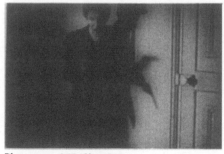

Photogram 277/Shot 221

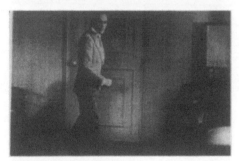

Photogram 278/Shot 222

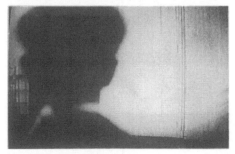

Photogram 279/Shot 223

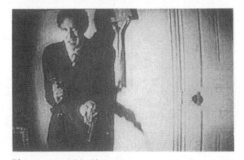

Photogram 280/Shot 224

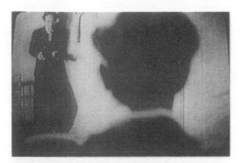

Photogram 281/Shot 225

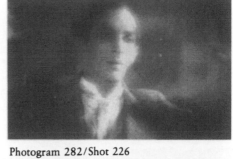

Photogram 282/Shot 226

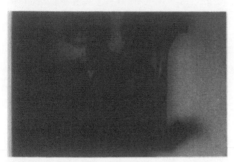

Photogram 283/Shot 227

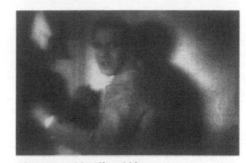

Photogram 284/Shot 228

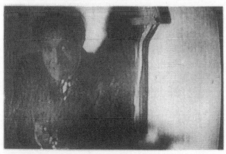

Photogram 285/Shot 229

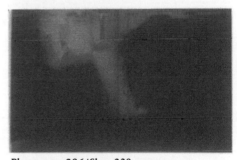

Photogram 286/Shot 230

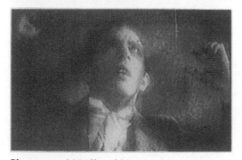

Photogram 287/Shot 231

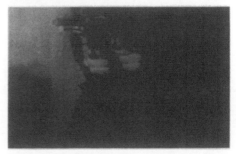

Photogram 288/Shot 232

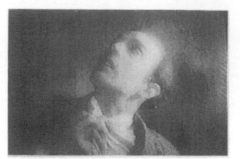

Photogram 289/Shot 233

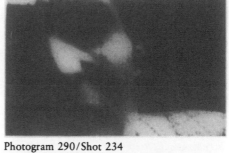

Photogram 290/Shot 234

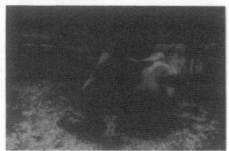

Photogram 291/Shot 235

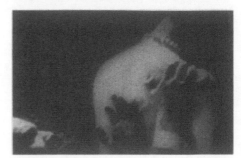

Photogram 292/Shot 236

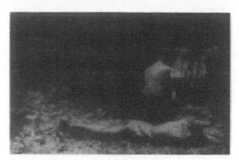

Photogram 293/Shot 237a

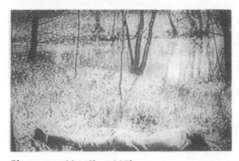

Photogram 294/Shot 237b

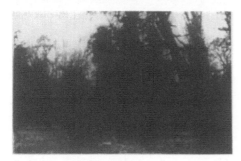

Photogram 295/Shot 238a

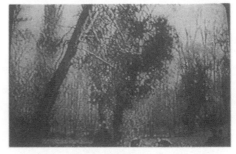

Photogram 296/Shot 238b

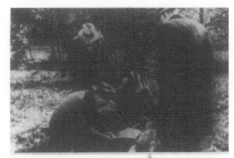

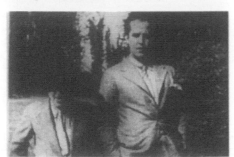

Photogram 297/Shot 239

Photogram 298/Shot 240

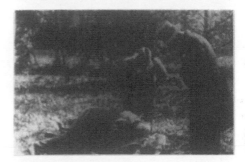

Photogram 299/Shot 241

Photogram 300/Shot 242

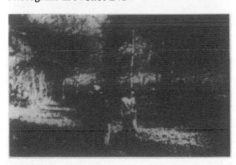

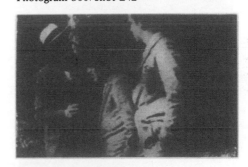

Photogram 301/Shot 243

Photogram 302/Shot 244

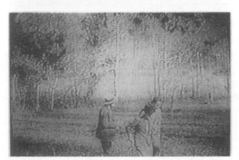

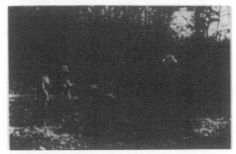

Photogram 303/Shot 245

Photogram 304/Shot 246a

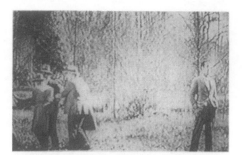

Photogram 305/Shot 246b

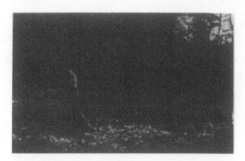

Photogram 306/Shot 246c

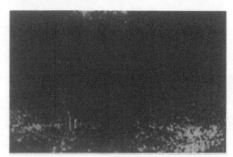

Photogram 307/Shot 247

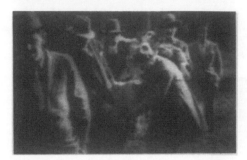

Photogram 308/Shot 248

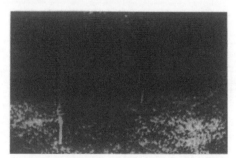

Photogram 309/Shot 249

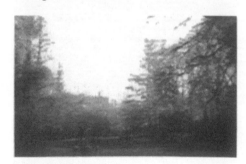

Photogram 310/Shot 250

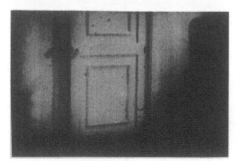

Photogram 311/Shot 251a

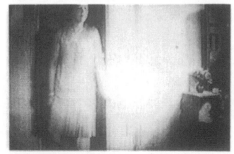

Photogram 312/Shot 251b

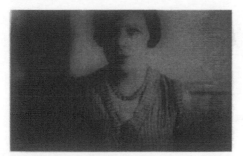

Photogram 313/Shot 252

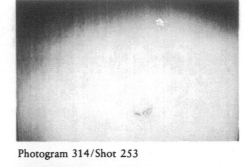

Photogram 314/Shot 253

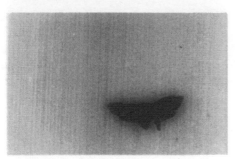

Photogram 315/Shot 254

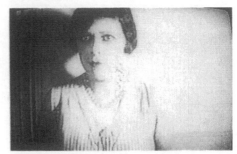

Photogram 316/Shot 255

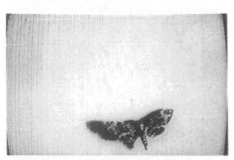

Photogram 317/Shot 256

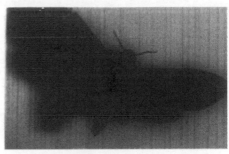

Photogram 318/Shot 257a

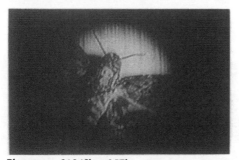

Photogram 319/Shot 257b

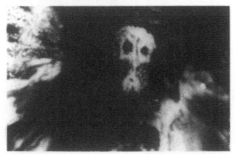

Photogram 320/Shot 258

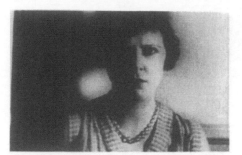

Photogram 321/Shot 259

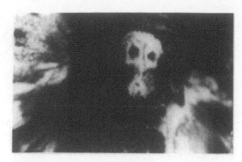

Photogram 322/Shot 260

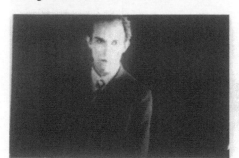

Photogram 323/Shot 261

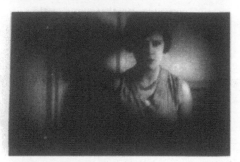

Photogram 324/Shot 262

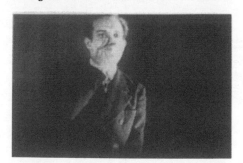

Photogram 325/Shot 263

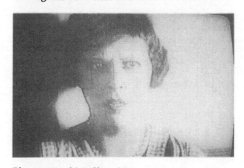

Photogram 326/Shot 264

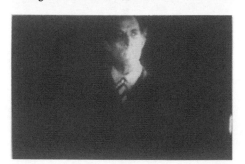

Photogram 327/Shot 265

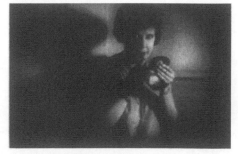

Photogram 328/Shot 266

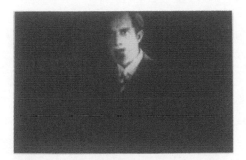

Photogram 329/Shot 267

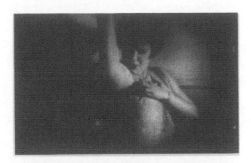

Photogram 330/Shot 268

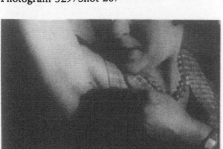

Photogram 331/Shot 269

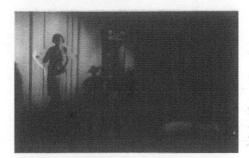

Photogram 332/Shot 270

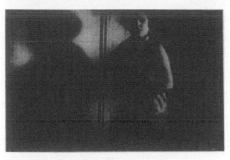

Photogram 333/Shot 271

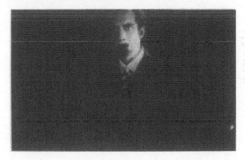

Photogram 334/Shot 272

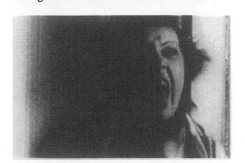

Photogram 335/Shot 273

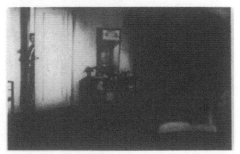

Photogram 336/Shot 274

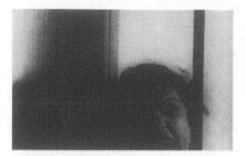

Photogram 337/Shot 275

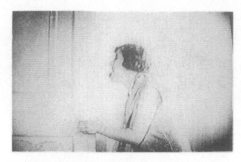

Photogram 338/Shot 276a

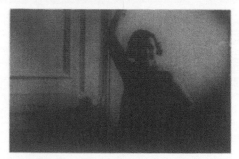

Photogram 339/Shot 276b

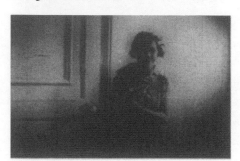

Photogram 340/Shot 277

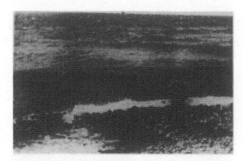

Photogram 341/Shot 278

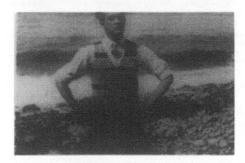

Photogram 342/Shot 279

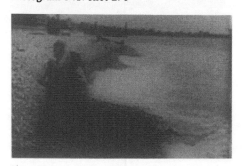

Photogram 343/Shot 280

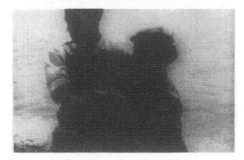

Photogram 344/Shot 281

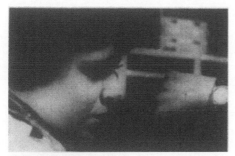

Photogram 345/Shot 282a

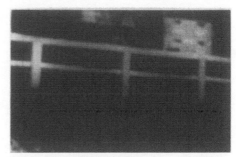

Photogram 346/Shot 282b

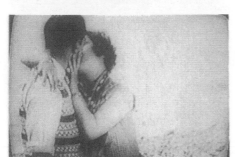

Photogram 347/Shot 283

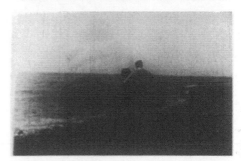

Photogram 348/Shot 284

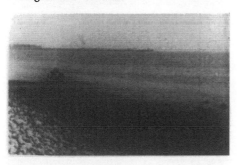

Photogram 349/Shot 285

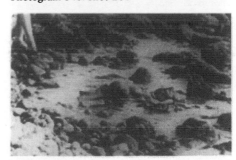

Photogram 350/Shot 286

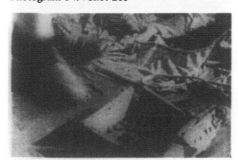

Photogram 351/Shot 287

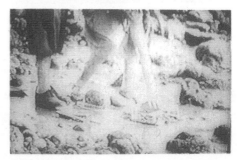

Photogram 352/Shot 288a

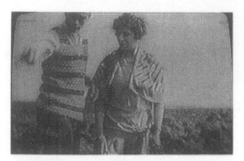

Photogram 353 / Shot 288b

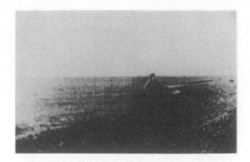

Photogram 354 / Shot 289

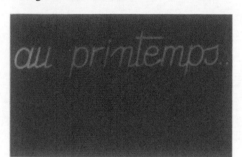

Photogram 355

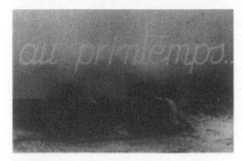

Photogram 356 / Shot 290a

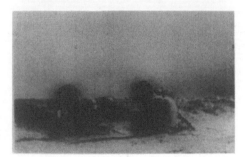

Photogram 357 / Shot 290b

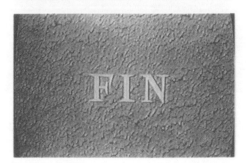

Photogram 358

Appendix 3
Film Synopsis

Un Chien andalou

Timing	Part	Segment	Span	Block	Intertitles	No.	Woman	Cyclist / Man / Double	Secondary	Tango 1	Tango 2	Wagner
00'00"		A			Sonorization credits							
00'02"										O¹		
00'26"		B			Film credits					O		
00'57"	1st	1	1–12	1st	Once upon a time	1	O		1. Man with the razor	O		
01'39"	2nd	2	13–21	1st	Eight years later.	2		O			O	
02'12"	2nd	3	22–49	1st			O	O	2. Pedestrians in the background			O
04'00"	2nd	4	50–58	2nd			O	O				O
04'21"	2nd	5	59–62	2nd					3. Swimmer's armpit			O
04'36"	2nd	6	63–99	2nd			O	O	4. Woman with severed hand 5. Policemen and crowd			O
06'24"	2nd	7	100–164	2nd			O	O	6. Pedestrians after the car crash 7. Marist brothers	O		O²
08'45"	2nd	8	165–170	3rd	About 3 A.M.	3	O	O		O	O	
09'19"	2nd	9	171–207	3rd			O	O			O	
10'46"	2nd	10	208–233	3rd	Sixteen years before.	4		O				O
12'04"	2nd	11	234–250	3rd			O	O	8. Men in the meadow			O
13'26"	2nd	12	251–276	4th			O			O		
14'21"	2nd	13	277–289	4th			O	O	9. Young man on the beach	O		
15'47"	3rd	14	290		In spring	5	O	O		O		
16'14"							O	O		O		

1. The music begins 2" after the first intertitle appears on the screen.
2. The Wagner music continues up to the middle of shot 105; tango no. 1 plays from the second half of shot 106 to the middle of shot 142; tango no. 2 begins from the middle of shot 144.

Notes

Introduction

1. On this topic see Conley (1988).

2. Even if the object of the present study is not film history per se, it may be relevant to cite some texts that have recently attempted to underscore the importance of film history for film theory: Heath (1981), Andrew (1983), Bordwell (1983), Thompson (1983), Bordwell et al. (1985). All of these texts take as point of departure film history as a theoretical object that preexists theoretical analysis. They do so from a standpoint influenced by Russian formalism (Bordwell, Thompson), by Althusserian postulates (Heath), or through the concept of figuration (Andrew). My view (Talens, 1989) is that film history, as object of an analysis that determines the inclusion or exclusion of films from the established canon and that hierarchizes directions, genres, or movements, can only be approached as the result of a previous theoretical construction. In this sense, the analysis of Buñuel's film would not so much look for its adequate place in film history as propose an alternative to the very notion of film history.

3. *The Kiss of Mary Pickford* (1925), made by a member of Kuleshov's collective, Serguei Komarov, is an excellent parodic example of how true this was even in Soviet Russia.

4. Juan-Miguel Company (1987) mentions that David W. Griffith, during his years at Biograph, defined himself as a Dickensian narrator who used the camera instead of a pen.

5. In recent years a representative of the so-called new avant-garde, Alexander Kluge, stated the following: "Film history seems to demonstrate that literary adaptations always have less to offer than literature. Looking at results alone — *these are two different media and for this reason their ability to produce expressive richness lies in different areas* — does not show the way out. One must above all go back to the common root of film and books: that is telling stories. People tell a story about something. They do this in an epic, a dramatic way, or in forms not specifically categorizable, always according to the circumstances. This is the *process*" (Kluge, 1983; cited in Rentschler, 1986, 1, emphasis in the original).

6. Pier Paolo Pasolini, "The Crisis of the Avant-Garde," in Louise K. Barnett, ed.,

171

Heretical Empiricism, trans. Ben Lawton and Louise K. Barnett (Bloomington, Ind.: Indiana University Press, 1988), 133.

1. Discursive Strategies and Production of Sense

1. An exception is Paul de Man (1979, 1983), whose work is as rigorous and incisive as Derrida's early work. Otherwise, those critics locating themselves openly on the side of what we could define, paraphrasing Geoffrey Hartman (1980), as "wild deconstruction," produce a sort of pseudowriting. Both for Hartman and for J. Hillis Miller (1970, 1977) interpretation is always submitted to an open chain of proliferating meanings that the critic can neither stop nor comprehend. Thus the critic can feel free to let his or her imagination loose when dealing with a specific text. See Christopher Norris (1982), Jonathan Arac et al. (1983), Tom Conley (1983), and Michael Fisher (1985). For a problematization of the relationship between deconstruction and Marxism, see Fredric Jameson (1981) and John Frow (1986).

2. In Lang's film *Fury* the reality effect of the institutional mode of representation is used to undo all elements of verisimilitude from within the logic of the plot. In fact, the proof used during the trial to prove the guilt of those implicated in the lynching of the main character (Spencer Tracy) is a documentary where impossible viewpoints and camera positions abound. Lang underscores the film's representational character from the very beginning by turning the court into a viewing room through the presence of a screen that a cut connects directly to the real screen showing *Fury* to the spectators in the movie theater. In the case of Sirk's film *All That Heaven Allows*, the story's credibility and the false happy ending as rhetorical effects have been discussed in depth and very poignantly by Jesús González-Requena (1986).

3. As we shall see later in our discussion of *Un Chien andalou*, Luis Buñuel had already criticized such function.

4. See the article I wrote in collaboration with Juan-Miguel Company at the time of the film's Spanish premiere, "En busca del objeto perdido."

5. Frank Tashlin did something similar with the studio's logo in *The Geisha Boy*, (1958). At one point in the film Jerry Lewis looks at a mountain far away on the horizon, and the circle of stars of the mountain of the logo of Paramount Pictures appears. In this case, however, the function is different, more subversive, if you will. The issue was to show how cinephilic education determines the way we look at films: cinema does not imitate reality; rather, reality reminds us of cinema.

6. Among them, first of all, Juan Ramón Jiménez, because of his association with the dead donkeys lying on the grand piano. The letter Buñuel and Dalí sent the poet is rather eloquent in this respect:

Distinguished friend: we feel it is our duty to let you know—
dispassionately—that we loathe your work for being immoral, hysteri-
cal, and arbitrary.

Especially: *MERDE!!* your *Platero & I*, your easy and ill-willed
Platero & I, the least donkey of all, the most hateful donkey we have ever
encountered.

SHIT!

Sincerely,

Luis Buñuel
Salvador Dalí

[Another English version of this text is found in Aranda (1976),
47.—Trans.]

7.   This explains the well-known anecdote about Buñuel in his Hollywood phase.
Buñuel stated that if one knew the characters' typologies and the film's initial
situation, one could come up with the story's development and end.

2. Reading of *Un Chien andalou*

1.   The recent rendering of the text by another megalomaniac who is also, though,
a much better director—Francis Ford Coppola—has proven that Buñuel was
right. Buñuel's rejection should not be considered, therefore, the act of youthful
rebellion against a man of the establishment; it was, rather, something much
more serious and motivated. By saying no to Gance, the Aragonese director was
saying no to a symbolist point of view, one dedicated to the search of "art."

2.   See his views on film collected in the documentary appendix of the volume edited by Rodolfo Cardona and Anthony N. Zahareas (1984).

3.   Each action or element is interpreted as having a very specific and unambiguous
meaning. The knife and the necktie represent the penis; the box represents the
vagina; and so on.

4.   Antonin Artaud was aware of the problem when, talking about Dulac's film,
he wondered "how far the scenario can resemble and ally itself with the me-
chanics of a dream without really being itself" (Artaud, *Collected Works*, 3:
63). See chapter 3 for a detailed analysis of the relationship between Artaud/
Dulac and Buñuel.

5.   See appendix 1 for a more detailed description of the sequences.

6.   See Cesarman (1976).

7.   In the shots where his face is visible, Buñuel wears an open shirt without a neck-

tie, and the hand holding the razor is the hand of someone wearing a necktie with diagonal stripes.

8. In *That Obscure Object of Desire*, the film that closes Buñuel's career as director, the character played by Fernando Rey (the actor that seems to function in Buñuel's films since *Tristana* as a sort of alter ego for the director, according to Buñuel's own words) has a similar function, even though, this time, from within the filmic discourse itself. The series of flashbacks articulating most of the story is justified only by the protagonist's desire to tell his story to his unknown but seemingly interested travel companions. In a more elaborate way, what they (and the spectators) see is not what the character played by Rey *sees*, but what *he says he sees*. Here the gaze is a product of listening, and the eye is a narrative construct. The authorial machinery dissolves in the filmic mechanisms, thus closing the circle.

9. In one of the best-known titles of the genre, *Deep Throat*, the director plays with this mechanism and makes explicit—with an irony rather unusual in this type of film—the workings of the so-called classical cinema. Thus the protagonist's orgasmic ecstasy is suggested by intercutting images of the sexual act with very short shots of a carillon's bronze statuettes hitting a bell, the launching of a rocket, and the explosion of fireworks in the night sky. This technique is also rather frequent in Alfred Hitchcock's films, as, for example, in the seduction scene between Cary Grant and Grace Kelly in the Côte d'Azur hotel room in *To Catch a Thief* (1954).

10. This is the reason why we can read the image of the man's hand with the ants crawling out of the hole in the middle of the palm as a masturbatory metaphor, corroborated by the series armpit-sea urchin-severed hand. This metaphor will appear again as a consequence of the woman's rejection of the man, whose hand is caught in the door after the sequence of the pianos.

11. See my quotation from "Caballería rusticana" in the next section of this chapter.

12. "Like the sea urchin, as you know, one day men got cold. And wanted to share it. Thus they invented love. The result was, as you know, as with the sea urchins." Parts of this long poem are available in Anthony Edkins et al., eds., *The Poetry of Luis Cernuda* (New York: New York University Press, 1971), 36–45.

13. Freudian psychoanalysis pointed out how the child's fear of losing the mother leads him or her to the accumulation of fetishes—plush toys, blankets (like the famous one of Linus), and so on—which, by substituting her absent presence through displacement, allows the acting out of incest via masturbation. This turns infantile onanism into a parallel form of either active voyeurism or passive exhibitionism, and may allow the explanation of the protagonist's fright in *Un Chien andalou* when he is caught in flagrante delicto by the "double" with all of his fetishes on top of him.

14. It is said that during the party given in Hollywood to celebrate the Academy Award won by Buñuel's *The Discreet Charm of the Bourgeoisie*, Alfred Hitchcock, present at the party with directors such as John Ford, William Wyler, and George Cukor, said about *Tristana*, "Ah! That leg, that leg!" Indeed, Buñuel's explicit perversion could not have escaped an old perversion-lover like Hitchcock.

15. See appendixes 1 and 2.

16. See note 6 of chapter 1. In the same way, Buñuel's scorn for Federico García Lorca's *The Love of Don Perlimplín and Belisa in the Garden* is cast in a new light from the weltanschauung at play in *Un Chien andalou*. (It is said that at a private reading the Andalusian poet gave of his text, Buñuel made the sharp remark, "You'd better leave it there, Federico; this is very bad.") The issue here is not Buñuel's lack of understanding of Lorca's text; what is at stake is rather two unreconcilable ways to look at reality. What in Lorca's text (whose value is undeniable) seems to result from the articulation of two elements understood as almost biological (women's attraction to change and an insurmountable age difference, the traditional topic of the young woman and the elder man) is, in Buñuel's work, the result of specific social and moral structures, which produce specific behaviors that are analyzable historically. What in Lorca takes as point of departure the notion of *discourse as representation*—what I have defined elsewhere as "writing as theatricality" (Talens, 1983)—gives way in Buñuel to the idea of *representation as discourse*. We can also note an allusion to Pepín Bello's "putrefied" in the image of the dead donkeys, an expression of Buñuel's rejection of the group's theoretical positions.

17. Like the notebook and the inkwell on the school desk, the moth also inscribes a reference that is perhaps comprehensible from within the universe of children's habits and games typical of Spanish society before the television age: the custom of growing silkworms. One of the mysteries of this strange breeding was the spectacle offered every fall and winter by each tiny worm's gradual transformation into a big one, the size of the little finger. At this point the caterpillar produced a silk thread in which it enveloped itself more and more until it disappeared inside the thread. A little later a moth emerged from the cocoon, similar to the one appearing in Buñuel's film. It died a few days later after laying a large amount of eggs, from which new caterpillars would be born the following autumn. The idea of death as transformation and not as just an end thus constituted a sort of counterpoint—not rationalized, albeit quite evident—to the imagery of suffering, pain, and loss associated with this concept in Catholic culture, which based even its most basic and simple rites on the sanctification of death.

18. See, for example, the following fragment from Aleixandre's poem "The Most Beautiful Love": "Faraway day before yesterday. / One very distant day / I met the glass I had never seen, / A butterfly made of tongue . . . / But I understood that everything was false. / False the manner of the cow dreaming / Of

being a pretty little budding virgin. / False the case of the false teacher who hoped, / In the end, to understand his nakedness. / False even the simple way girls / At night hang up their untouched breasts" [in *Swords like Lips*, in Vicente Aleixandre, *The Crackling Sun: Selected Poems of the Nobel Prize Recipient, 1977*, trans. Louis Bourne (Alcobendas, Spain: Sociedad General Española de Libreria, 1981), 106].

19. The topic of Millet's *Angelus*, one of Dalí's favorites and about which the painter would later write a book, is a recurring theme in Buñuel as well. It appears in *Belle de jour* (1966) in a strange scene in which Pierre and Hudson stand, like the farmers in Millet's painting, as some bulls appear in the background. Pierre asks Hudson, "Do bulls have a name, like cats?" Hudson replies: "They do. Most of them are called Remorse, except for the last one, whose name is Expiation."

20. The theme of *The Lacemaker* and of the young lady that spins, sews, or embroiders appears in many of Buñuel's films associated to the theme of infidelity. See, for example, *La mort dans ce jardin* or *Belle de jour*. In *That Strange Passion* this theme appears anecdotically paraphrased when the main character, paranoically jealous of his wife, attempts to sew her genitals while she sleeps. In *Viridiana* the title character throws knitting needles and wool into the fire as a prelude to her forsaking the convent, (see Sánchez-Vidal, 1988). In Buñuel's last film, *That Obscure Object of Desire*, the image of the lacemaker appears explicitly in the film's final sequence, the last one the director shot before his death; as in *Un Chien andalou*, it is associated with the main characters' impossibility for sexual fulfillment, as Mathieu (Fernando Rey) and Conchita (Carole Bouquet) contemplate the lacemaker through a shop window.

21. Cesarman (1976) noted that a peculiar feature in Buñuel's filmography is the absence of the mother figure (except for the mother as victim in *Susana* or as victimizer in *The Young and the Damned*), as well as the lack of direct references to homosexuality and to the topic of women's liberation, despite the importance of these issues in the cinema of his time. That such issues are not part of his films' subject matter, however, does not mean that the problematic they imply is not present. The choice of the woman's point of view as articulator of the discourse of *Un Chien andalou* is, at least by its being there if not in its direct implications, a clear sign of a will to not elude the problem. A different question is how the problem is (not) resolved.

22. See the difference in tone between the virulence of this fragment and the decadent lyricism with which Lorca confronted a similar topic in *Doña Rosita, the Spinster, or The Language of the Flowers*.

23. These fragments were written in 1927. A different English translation of these texts (as "A Proper Story" and "An Improper Story") appears in Aranda (1976), 256–57.

24. Emilio Sanz de Soto, Buñuel's friend and occasional collaborator, told me a

funny anecdote in this regard about the editing of *Diary of a Chambermaid*. It seems that Buñuel did not want such an "experienced" and "famous" actress as Jeanne Moreau to play the part; eventually he accepted her because of the great interest the actress showed in working with him. During the shooting of a sequence, Moreau asked him whether she should concentrate on the object as she picked up a glass, or whether, on the contrary, what mattered was her expression of disconcertedness as she picked up the glass thoughtlessly. Buñuel turned to his assistant director with an astonished expression on his face and said laconically: "We have just screwed up the film." The actress won the first prize at the Karlóvy Váry Festival in 1964 for her role in the film.

25. Quite curiously, this passage by Wagner has constituted a leitmotiv in Buñuel's filmography, where music is generally rarely used, unless imposed by the production regimen. Rather than music, Buñuel preferred noise or a "sonorous background" prepared by himself.

26. The same topic articulates, although in a simpler way, *Last Tango in Paris* (Bernardo Bertolucci, 1972), in which the love story ends exactly when the so-far anonymous male character (Marlon Brando) finds an identity in a name, age, and so on; that is, when he attempts to become part of the space of a relationship acknowledged by the law and the social order.

3. A Writing of Disorder

1. See Steven Kovacs (1980), Linda Williams (1981), Inez Hedges (1983), Richard Abel (1984), Naomi Greene (1984), and Sandy Flitterman-Lewis (1984, 1986). Artaud (1972) translates the title of this work as *The Shell and the Clergyman*; this title will be used when referring to quotations from this translation.

2. Besides *The Seashell and the Clergyman*, Artaud wrote six screenplays that were never shot: *Eighteen Seconds, Two Nations on the Borders of Mongolia . . . , Thirty-Two, The Butcher's Revolt, Flights*, and *The Master of Ballantrae*. Also, there is a fragment of an eighth screenplay and another one, *Le bon sens*, that is signed with his name but whose paternity seems unclear. The author of that text probably is Mme Allendy.

3. In the copy in Super 8 of the film that I am using as a referent, there is only an intertitle with the title of the film, the date (1928), and the indication: "réalisé par Germaine Dulac." The name of Antonin Artaud is not credited. It is known that the assistant director was Louis Ronjat, the photographer was Paul Guichard, and the roles of the woman, the clergyman, and the official were performed, respectively, by Génica Athanasiou, Alex Allin, and Georges Bataille.

4. The explicit affirmation by Artaud was that there was not a "hidden meaning" in the images of his film.

5. In effect, some of the surrealist texts make continuous reference to the writers'

own past, or to the place where they locate the story they are narrating, such as the Paris of the "Passage de l'Opéra" in *Le Paysan de Paris* by Louis Aragon or the Paris of theaters to which Breton alludes in *Nadja*.

6. See the découpage of the film in Conley (1988).

7. The translation of "No me parece bien ni mal" is by the translator of this book; this fragment of "Bird of Anguish" appears in Aranda (1976), 261.

8. From Georges Bataille, *Theory of Religion*, trans. Robert Hurley (New York: Zone Books, 1989), 9.

Appendix 1: Script and Description of the Découpage of *Un Chien andalou*

1. There is no rain in the finished film; we see only a slightly wet ground. Also, the man's hands do hold the handlebars of the bicycle in the film.

2. In the film there is neither a gutter nor mud.

3. This indication was not followed in the film.

4. See note 1.

5. In the film only the pillow is slightly rumpled.

6. The sea urchin does not move in the film.

7. In the film the fingernails are not painted.

8. In the film the girl makes no move to a gesture of thanks; she remains as absent as in the rest of the sequence.

9. This indication was not followed in the film. The two people do not cry out and do not make any nodding movement.

10. This indication was not followed in the film. We only see her body lying on the street in a long high-angle shot.

11. This indication was not followed in the film, where the woman's breasts remain offscreen.

12. Buttocks appear in the film instead of thighs.

13. In the film the order is reversed: first she breaks away from his hold and then she runs to the middle of the room.

14. A chair in the film.

15. The standard English version of the script replaces "her aggressor" with "he." — TRANS.

16. In the film there is neither the cork nor the melon, but two wide corkboards. Their shape recalls the tables of law that appeared in the *Sacred History* books used in the Marist brothers' schools. The man does not knock anything down. The rumps of the donkeys do not get caught in anything. The light does not rock from side to side. [The standard English version of the script translates erroneously "Hermanos de las escuelas cristianas" as "Catholic priests." "Hermanos" (brothers) are not priests: they cannot celebrate. Secondly, "escuelas cristianas" describes a specific kind of private religious school. All religious schools in Spain were "Catholic."—TRANS.]

17. His arm is caught at the elbow in the film.

18. In the film the ants do not crawl out of the man's hand.

19. In the original script: "Unlike in mainstream films"—TRANS.

20. In the film we see two arms dressed in white.

21. I do not know what Buñuel and Dalí meant with "moral meaning" when they talk about the objects' position on the school desk. In any case, if they allude to the rigidity with which order and cleanness were imposed on young students in Marist brothers' schools, the film shows just the opposite: disorder and filth. [This note is based on the description that appears in the original script. The English translation renders with "the placing of the objects must have a clear and symbolic meaning," what in the Spanish text used by the author sounds more like: "the placing of the objects and their moral meaning have to be determined carefully."—TRANS.]

22. This is the only shot where the two men, played by the same actor (Pierre Batcheff) when facing each other, both appear in the same frame. The vertical line of the door crossbar has very likely allowed the fusion in one frame of two separately shot half-frames. In effect the shot ends precisely when the hands of man no. 2 extend forward and reach the crossbar.

23. Neither a lame nor a passionate man is in the sequence. It may be of interest to note that from his very first film Buñuel associates eroticism and cruelty with people marked by some physical impairment (people who are blind, maimed, lame, crippled, and so on). *The Age of Gold*, *The Young and the Damned*, *Viridiana*, and *Tristana* show examples of this association. [The standard English version of the script translates this annotation as if it had been actually shot: "just as a lame man comes into shot."—TRANS.]

24. This shot is missing from the film; there is a cut to the moth sequence.

25. It only covers the middle section of the frame in the film.

26. In the film she drops the powder compact and the lipstick first.

27. The order is reversed in the film: first she throws a shawl over her shoulders and then sticks out her tongue.

28. The film first shows a little quarrel because of the woman's delay, and there are no waves, but a quiet sea. [As in note 21, this note refers to the Spanish script; the English "following the shoreline" translates the Spanish "al borde del oleaje," which should be rendered with "along the waves."—TRANS.]

29. In the film the objects are already lying on the beach, except for the bicycle, which we never see.

30. The insects do not appear in the film; the man and the woman do not wear rags; and more than by a devouring sun, they are covered by a grayish and dull light.

Bibliography

Abel, Richard. 1984. *French Cinema: The First Wave, 1915–1929*. Princeton: Princeton University Press.

Abruzzese, Alberto, and Stefano Masi. 1981. *I films di Luis Buñuel*. Rome: Gremese.

Agel, Henry. 1959. *Luis Buñuel*. Paris: Ed. Universitaires.

Alcalá, Manuel. 1973. *Buñuel: cine e ideología*. Madrid: Editorial Cuadernos para el diálogo.

Andrew, Dudley. 1983. "On Figuration." *Iris* 1 (January-March).

Arac, J., W. Godzich, and W. Martin, ed. 1983. *The Yale Critics: Deconstruction in America*. Minneapolis: University of Minnesota Press.

Aranda, José Francisco. 1953. *Cinema de vanguardia en España*. Lisbon: Guimarães.

——. 1959. "Buñuel." *Cinema Universitario* (Salamanca) 4.

——. 1961. "Surrealistic and Spanish Giant." *Film and Filming* (October).

——. 1969. *Luis Buñuel, biografía crítica*. Barcelona: Editorial Lumen. [*Luis Buñuel: A Critical Biography*. Trans. and ed. David Robinson. New York: Da Capo Press, 1976.]

Armes, Roy. 1974. "Buñuel and Surrealism." In *Film and Reality*. London: Penguin Books.

Artaud, Antonin. 1976. *Oeuvres Complètes*. 5 vols. Paris: Gallimard. [*Collected Works*. 5 vols. Trans. Alastair Hamilton. London: Calder & Boyars, 1972.]

Aub, Max. 1985. *Conversaciones con Buñuel*. Madrid: Aguilar.

Barthes, Roland. 1966. "Introduction." In *L'analyse structural du récit, Communication*.

——. 1970. "Le troisième sens: Notes de recherche sur quelques photogrammes de S. M. Eisenstein." *Cahiers du Cinéma* 222.

——. 1973. *Le plaisir du texte*. Paris: Seuil. [*The Pleasure of the Text*. Trans. R. Miller. New York: Hill and Wang, 1975.]

Baudry, Jean-Louis. 1970. "Cinéma: Effets idéologiques produits par l'appareil de base." *Cinéthique* 7–8.

Bazin, André. 1962. "The Depths of Reality." In Ado Kyrou, *Luis Buñuel: An Introduction*. Trans. Adrienne Foulke. New York: Simon & Schuster, 1963. 189–92.

Bernadi, Auro. 1984. *L'arte dello scandalo*. Bari, Italy: Edizioni Dedalo.

Bobker, Lee R. 1969. *Elements of Film*. New York: Harcourt Brace & World.

Bordwell, David. 1983. "Lowering the Stakes: Prospects for a Historical Poetics of Cinema." *Iris* 1 (January-March): 5–18.

———, Janet Steiger, and Kristin Thompson. 1985. *The Classical Hollywood Cinema: Film Style and Mode of Production to 1960.* New York: Columbia University Press.

Bragaglia, Cristina. 1975. *La realità dell'immagine in Luis Buñuel.* Bologna: Patron.

Branigan, Edward. 1975. "Formal Permutations of the Point-of-View Shot." *Screen* 16: 54–64.

Breton, André. 1969. "Manifesto of Surrealism." In *Manifestoes of Surrealism.* Trans. Richard Seaver and Helen R. Lane. Ann Arbor, Mich.: University of Michigan Press. 3–47.

Browne, Nick. 1975. "The Spectator-in-the-Text: The Rhetoric of *Stagecoach*." *Film Quarterly* 29: 26–38.

Brunius, Jacques B. 1929. "*Un Chien andalou*: A Poet's Lucidity." In Ado Kyrou, *Luis Buñuel: An Introduction.* Trans. Adrienne Foulke. New York: Simon & Schuster, 1963. 181.

Bruno, Edoardo. 1963. "La poetica di Buñuel." *Filmcritica* 130.

Buache, Freddy. 1960. "Luis Buñuel." *Premier Plan* (Serdoc, Lyon) 13.

———. 1970. *Luis Buñuel.* Lausanne: Ed. La Cité.

Buñuel, Luis. 1968. *L'Age d'Or and Un Chien andalou.* Classic Film Scripts. Trans. Marianne Alexandre. Letchworth, Hertfordshire: Lorrimer.

———. 1984. *My Last Sigh: The Autobiography of Luis Buñuel.* Trans. Abigail Israel. New York: Vintage Books.

Burch, Noël. 1981. *Theory of Film Practice.* Trans. Helen R. Lane. Princeton: Princeton University Press. [Original French edition: *Praxis du Cinéma*, 1969.]

———. 1984. *Itinerarios.* Ed. Santos Zunzunegui. Bilbao, Spain: Publicaciones del Festival Internacional de Cine de Bilbao.

———. 1987. *El tragaluz del infinito.* Trans. Francisco Llinás. Madrid: Ediciones Cátedra. [*Life to Those Shadows.* Trans. and ed. Ben Brewster. London: BFI, 1990.]

———, and Jorge Dana. 1974. "Propositions." *Afterimage 5.*

Cappabianca, Alessandro. 1972. "Film: Segni e Strutture." In Galvano della Volpe et al., *Teoria e prassi del cinema in Italia 1950–1970.* Milan: Mazzotta.

Cardona, Rodolfo, and Anthony N. Zahareas. 1984. *Visión del esperpento.* 2d ed. Madrid: Castalia.

Casiraghi, Ugo. 1966. *Il diabolico Buñuel.* Imola, Italy: Filmquaderni del Circolo del Cinema di Imola.

Cattini, Alberto. 1979. *Luis Buñuel.* Florence: Il Castoro Cinema, La Nuova Italia.

Cavell, Stanley. 1971. *The World Viewed: Reflections on the Ontology of Film.* New York: Viking Press.

Cesarman, Fernando. 1976. *El ojo de Buñuel: psicoanálisis desde una butaca.* Barcelona: Anagrama.

Colina, José de la. 1980. "El cuchillo espectral." *Contracampo* (Madrid) 16.

———, and Tomás Pérez Turrent. 1980. "Entrevista con Luis Buñuel." *Contracampo* (Madrid) 16.

Company, Juan-Miguel. 1978. "El ghetto pornográfico." *La Mirada*, (Madrid) 1.

———. 1983. "Perro ladrador." *Contracampo* (Madrid) 33.

———. 1986. *La realidad como sospecha.* Valencia and Madrid: Eutopías/Hiperión.

——. 1987. *El trazo de la letra en la imagen*. Madrid: Ediciones Cátedra.
——, and Julio Pérez Perucha. 1983. "Dalí y el cine. Luis Buñuel." *Contracampo* (Madrid) 33.
——, and Jenaro Talens. 1981. "En busca del objeto perdido." *Contracampo* (Madrid) 25–26: 64–67.
——, and ——. 1984. "The Textual Space: 'On the Notion of Text.'" *MMLA* 17, no. 2.
Conley, Tom. 1983. "A Trace of Style." In Mark Krupnick, ed., *Displacement: Derrida and After*. Bloomington, Ind.: Indiana University Press. 74–92.
——. 1988. *Su realismo. Lectura de "Tierra sin pan."* Valencia: Fundación Instituto Shakespeare, *Documentos de trabajo* 6.
Conrad, Randall. 1974. *Luis Buñuel: Surrealist and Filmmaker*. Boston: Museum of Modern Art (mimeograph).
——. 1976. " 'The Minister of the Interior Is on the Telephone'—The Early Films of Luis Buñuel." *Cineaste* 7, no. 3.
Cremoni, Giorgio. 1973. *Buñuel*. Rome: Savelli.
Dalí, Salvador. 1935. *The Conquest of the Irrational*. New York: Julien Levy.
——. 1942. *The Secret Life of Salvador Dalí*. Trans. Haakon M. Chevalier. New York: Dial Press.
——. 1955. "Comments on the Making of *Un Chien andalou*." *Cinemages* (New York) 1: 25–27.
de Man, Paul. 1979. *Allegories of Reading: Figural Language in Rousseau, Nietzsche, Rilke and Proust*. New Haven, Conn.: Yale University Press.
——. 1983. *Blindness and Insight*. 2d ed. Minneapolis: University of Minnesota Press.
Drouzy, Maurice. 1978. *Luis Buñuel architecte du rêve*. Paris: L'herminier.
Drummond, Phillip. 1977. "Textual space in *Un Chien andalou*." *Screen* 18, no. 3: 55–119.
Dufrenne, Mikel. 1979. *Subversion/Perversion*. Paris: PUF.
Dulac, Germaine. 1925. "L'essence du cinéma, l'idée visuelle." *Les Cahiers du Mois* 16/17. ["The Essence of the Cinema: The Visual Idea," in P. Adams Sitney, ed., *The Avant-Garde Film: A Reader of Theory and Criticism* (New York: New York University Press, 1978), 36–42.]
——. 1928. "La musique du silence." *Cinégraphie* 5 (15 January).
Durgnat, Raymond. 1962. "Erotism in Cinema." *Film and Filming* 7.
——. 1967. *Luis Buñuel*. London: Studio Vista. [Revised ed., Berkeley: University of California Press, 1977.]
Edwards, Gwynne. 1982. *The Discreet Art of Luis Buñuel*. London and Boston: Marion Boyars.
Esteve, Michel, ed. 1962 and 1963. *Luis Buñuel. Etudes Cinématographiques* 20–21 and 22–23.
Ferrero, Adelio. 1971. *Buñuel: continuità di una rivolta*. Modena, Italy: Quaderni del Circolo Cabassi.
——. 1978. "La rivoluzione surrealista e il primo Buñuel." In Adelio Ferrero, ed., *Storia del cinema*, vol. 1. Venice: Marsilio.
Fink, Guido. 1966. *Luis Buñuel. Documenta*. Genova: Quaderni del CUC.

Fisher, Michael. 1985. *Does Deconstruction Make Any Difference? Post-structuralism and the Defense of Poetry in Modern Criticism.* Bloomington, Ind.: Indiana University Press.

Flitterman-Lewis, Sandy. 1984. "The Feminine: Woman as the Figure of Desire in *The Seashell and the Clergyman.*" *Wide Angle* 6: 3.

———. 1986. "The Image and the Spark: Dulac and Artaud Reviewed." *Dada/Surrealism* 15: 110–27.

Frow, John. 1986. *Marxism and Literary History.* Oxford: Basil Blackwell.

Fuentes, Carlos. 1976. "Prólogo." In Fernando Cesarman, *El ojo de Buñuel: psicoanálisis desde una butaca.* Barcelona: Anagrama.

Gálvez, Antonio. 1970. *Luis Buñuel.* Paris: Le Terrain Vague.

García, Germán L. 1983. *Psicoanálisis dicho de otra manera.* Valencia: Pretextos.

Garroni, Emilio. 1974. *Proyecto de semiótica.* Barcelona: Gustavo Gili.

———. 1979. *Ricognizione della semiotica.* Bari, Italy: Laterza.

Goetz, Alice, and Helmut Banz. 1965. *Luis Buñuel, eine Dokumentation.* Bad Ems: Verband der Deuschen Film-clubs.

González-Requena, Jesús. 1986. *La metáfora del espejo. El cine de Douglas Sirk.* Valencia and Madrid: Eutopías/Hiperión.

Goudal, Jean. 1925. "Surréalisme et cinéma." *Révue hebdomadaire 34*, no. 8 (21 February 1925): 343–57. [For English translation, see Paul Hammond, *The Shadow and Its Shadow: Surrealist Writings on Cinema* (London: British Film Institute, 1978), 49–56.]

Gould, Michael. 1976. "Luis Buñuel." In *Surrealism and the Cinema.* London: The Tantivy Press.

Greene, Naomi. 1984. "Artaud and Film: A Reconsideration." *Cinema Journal* 23: 4.

Hartman, Geoffrey. 1980. *Criticism in Wilderness.* New Haven, Conn.: Yale University Press.

Heath, Stephen. 1981. *Questions of Cinema.* Bloomington, Ind.: Indiana University Press.

———, and Gillian Skirrow. 1977. "Television: A World in Action." *Screen* 18, no. 2: 7–59.

Hedges, Inez. 1983. *Languages of Revolt: Dada and Surrealist Literature and Film.* Durham N.C.: Duke University Press.

Higginbotham, Virginia. 1979. *Luis Buñuel.* Twayne's Theatrical Arts Series. Boston: Twayne Publishers.

Jameson, Fredric. 1981. *The Political Unconscious.* London: Methuen.

Kermode, Frank. 1966. *The Sense of an Ending.* London: Oxford University Press.

Kluge, Alexander. 1983. *Bestandsaufnahme: Utopie Film.* Frankfurt am Main: Zweitausendeins.

Kovacs, Steven. 1980. *From Enchantment to Rage.* London and Toronto: Associated University Presses.

Kovacs, Yves, ed. 1965. *Surréalisme et Cinéma. Études Cinématographiques.* Vols. 38–39, 40–42.

Kristeva, Julia. 1987. *Tales of Love.* Trans. Leon S. Roudiez. New York: Columbia

University Press. [Original French edition: *Histories d'amour*. Paris: Denoel, 1983.]

Kuntzel, Thierry. 1972. "Le Travail du Film." *Communications* 19.

———. 1975. "Le Travail du Film, 2." *Communications* 23.

Kyrou, Ado. 1953. "Luis Buñuel." In *Le surréalisme au cinema*. Paris: Arcanes. Revised ed., Ramsey, 1985. 207–68.

———. 1963. *Luis Buñuel: An Introduction*. Trans. Adrienne Foulke. New York: Simon & Schuster.

Lara, Antonio, ed. 1981. *La imaginación en libertad (homenaje a Luis Buñuel)*. Madrid: Universidad Complutense.

Lefevre, Raymond. 1984. *Luis Buñuel*. Paris: Edilig.

Lerg, Winfried B. 1960. "Vivisektion des Auges." *Filmforum* 8–9.

Lizalde, Eduardo. 1962. "Luis Buñuel: odisea del demoledor." *Cuadernos de Cine*, vol. 2. Mexico City: Universidad Autónoma de México.

Lozano, J., C. Peña-Marin, and G. Abril. 1982. *Análisis del discurso*. Madrid: Ediciones Cátedra.

Malerba, Luigi. 1949. "Un Chien andalou." *Cinema* 19.

Mareschal, Gilbert. 1958–59. "Le rasoir émoussé." *Film Klub/Ciné-Club* (Zurich and Geneva) 12.

Marie, Michel. 1977. "Muet." In Jean Collet et al., eds., *Lectures du film*. Paris: Albatros.

Mariniello, Silvestra. 1989. *Lev Kuleshov*. Milan: Il Castoro, La Nuova Italia.

———. 1992. *El cine y el fin del arte. Teoría y práctica cinematográfica en Lev Kuleshov*. Trans. Anna Giordano and Ponzio Almodóvar. Madrid: Ediciones Cátedra.

Masterman, Len. 1970. "*Cul-de-sac*: Through the Mirror of Surrealism." *Screen* 11, no. 6: 44–60.

Matthews, J. 1971. *Surrealism and Film*. Ann Arbor, Mich.: University of Michigan Press.

Mellen, Joan, ed. 1978. *The World of Luis Buñuel: Essays in Criticism*. New York: Oxford University Press.

Miller, Henry. 1939. "The Golden Age." In *The Cosmological Eye*. New York: New Directions. Reprinted in Daniel Talbot, ed., *Film: An Anthropology*. New York: Simon & Schuster, 1959. 498–509.

Miller, J. Hillis. 1970. *Thomas Hardy: Distance and Desire*. Cambridge, Mass.: Harvard University Press.

———. 1977. "The Limits of Pluralism, II: The Critic as Host." *Critical Inquiry* 3: 439–47.

Mondragon. 1949. "Comment j'ai compris *Un Chien andalou*." *Ciné-club* 8–9.

Monterde, José Enrique, and Esteve Riambau. 1979. "Cine y surrealismo." *Dirigido por* (Barcelona) 64.

Morris, C. B. 1972. *Surrealism and Spain: 1920–1936*. Cambridge: Cambridge University Press.

Moullet, Luc. 1957. *Luis Buñuel*. Club du livre du cinéma, vol. 5. Brussels: Collection Encyclopédique du Cinéma.

Norris, Christopher. 1982. *Deconstruction: Theory and Practice*. London and New York: Methuen.

Noszlopy, George T. 1969. "The Embourgeoisement of Avant-garde Art." *Diógenes* 67.

Oms, Marcel. 1961. "Luis Buñuel." *Positif* 42.

———. 1985. *Don Luis Buñuel*. Paris: Les éditions du Cerf.

Paz, Octavio. 1951. "The Tradition of a Fierce and Passionate Art." In Ado Kyrou, *Luis Buñuel: An Introduction*. Trans. Adrienne Foulke. New York: Simon & Schuster, 1963. 186–89.

———. 1964. *Cuadrivio*. Mexico City: Joaquín Mortiz.

———. 1971. *Los hijos del limo*. Barcelona: Seix Barral.

Perrier, Jean-Louis. 1969. "L'oeil tranché." *Cinéthique* 7–8.

Phillippe, Jean-Claude. 1960. "Luis Buñuel du *Chien andalou* à *Nazarín*." *Télérama* 18.

Piazza, François. 1949. "Considération psychanalitique sur *Un Chien andalou*." *Psyché*.

Poggioli, Renato. 1968. *The Theory of the Avant-Garde*. Trans. Gerald Fitzgerald. Cambridge, Mass.: Harvard University Press.

Polan, Dana Bart. 1985. *The Political Language of Film and the Avant-Garde*. Ann Arbor, Mich.: University of Michigan Research Press.

Pornon, Charles. 1959. *L'écran merveilleux*. Paris: La Nef.

Ramsey, Cynthia. 1983. *The Problem of Dual Consciousness: The Structures of Dream and Reality in the Films of Luis Buñuel*. Ann Arbor, Mich.: University Microfilm International.

Rebolledo, Carlos, and Frederic Grange. 1964. *Luis Buñuel*. Paris: Ed. Universitaires.

Renan, Sheldon. 1968. *An Introduction to the American Underground Film*. London: Studio Vista.

Rentschler, Eric, ed. 1986. *German Film and Literature: Adaptations and Transformations*. London: Methuen.

Ribemont-Dessaignes, Georges. 1973. *Déjà-jadis ou du Mouvement Dada à l'espace abstrait*. Paris: René Julliard.

Risi, Nelo. 1962. "Buñuel o il sogno della ragione." *L'Europa letteraria* 15–16.

Rondolino, Gianni. 1972. *L'occhio tagliato*. Turin: Martano.

Russell, Charles. 1985. *Poets, Prophets and Revolutionaries: The Literary Avant-Garde from Rimbaud through Postmodernism*. New York: Oxford University Press.

Sadoul, Georges. 1965. "Souvenirs d'un Témoin." *Études Cinématographiques* 38–39.

Sánchez-Vidal, Agustín, ed. 1982. *Luis Buñuel. Obra literaria*. Zaragoza: Ediciones del Heraldo de Aragón.

———. 1984. *Luis Buñuel. Obra cinematográfica*. Madrid: Ediciones J. C.

———. 1988. *Buñuel, Lorca, Dalí: el enigma sin fin*. Barcelona: Planeta.

Sandro, Paul. 1981. "The Management of Destiny in Narrative Form." *Cine-Tracts* 4: 50–56.

———. 1987. *Diversions of Pleasure: Luis Buñuel and the Crisis of Desire.* Columbus, Ohio: Ohio State University Press.

Schwarze, Michael. 1981. *Buñuel.* Hamburg: Taschenbuch Verlag GMBH.

Seguin, Louis. 1962. "En attendant Buñuel." *Positif* 47.

Soriano, Marc. 1946. "Le Surréalisme au cinéma." *Formes et couleurs* 6.

Stam, Robert. 1989. *Subversive Pleasures: Bakhtin, Cultural Criticism, and Film.* Baltimore: The Johns Hopkins University Press.

Stauffacher, Frank. 1947. *Notes on the Making of* Un Chien andalou: *Cinema.* San Francisco: Museum of Modern Art.

Talens, Jenaro. 1975. *El espacio y las máscaras. Introducción a la lectura de Cernuda.* Barcelona: Anagrama.

———. 1983. *El discurso poético lorquiano: medievalismo y teatralidad.* Granada: Editorial Don Quijote.

———. 1985. "Documentalidad *vs.* Ficcionalidad." *Revista de Occidente* (Madrid) 53.

———. 1987. "Was as Pretext: The Referential Effect." MMLA Annual Meeting, Columbus, Ohio (mimeograph).

———. 1989. "La storia del cinema come invenzione della teoria filmica." Convegno su storia del cinema, Urbino, Italy (mimeograph).

Thompson, Kristin. 1983. "Cinematic Specificity in Film Criticism and History." *Iris* 1 (January-March): 39–49.

Tinazzi, Giorgio. 1973. *Il cinema di Luis Buñuel.* Palermo, Italy: Palumbo.

Trebouta, Jacques. 1958–59. *Luis Buñuel, sa vie, son oeuvre en Espagne et en France.* Paris: Institut des Hautes Études Cinématographiques.

Verdone, Mario. 1977. *Le avanguardie storiche del cinema.* Turin: SEI.

Virmaux, Alain and Odette. 1976. *Les surrealistes et le cinéma.* Paris: Seghers.

Williams, Linda. 1981. *Figures of Desire: A Theory and Analysis of Surrealist Film.* Chicago: University of Illinois Press.

The following list is a selection of monographic issues that are studies of Buñuel and his cinema.

Luis Buñuel. Filme Culture 21 (1960).

Luis Buñuel. Cinema 60 23–26 (1962).

Luis Buñuel. La Méthode 7 (1962).

Luis Buñuel. Image et Son 157 (1962).

Pour Buñuel. Toulouse: Cercle du Cinéma de l'A.C.E.T. (1964).

Luis Buñuel. Positif 58 (1964).

Luis Buñuel. La Nouvelle Critique 57–58 (1972).

Saggi e studi su Buñuel. Cinema Nuovo 227 (1974).

Luis Buñuel tra surrealismo e industria culturale. Cinema e Cinema 4 (1975).

Luis Buñuel. Contracampo 16 (1980).

Le cinéma des surréalistes. Les Cahiers de la Cinémathèque 30–31 (1980).

Surréalisme et cinéma. Jeune Cinéma 134 (1981).

Luis Buñuel. Lisbon: Cinemateca Portuguesa (1982).

Dossier: Luis Buñuel. Cinématographe 92 (1983).

Luis Buñuel: A Symposium. Trinity and all Saints College (1983).

Index

Compiled by Robin Jackson

Jenaro Talens is professor of literary theory and film at the University of Valencia. He has written fifteen books of poetry and has published widely on literary theory and history. Among his publications are *Romanticism and the Writing of Modernity* (1989) and, with Nicholas Spadaccini, *Through the Shattering Glass: Cervantes and the Self-Made World* (Minnesota, 1992).

Giulia Colaizzi holds a doctorate in English from the University of Valencia, Spain, and is a doctoral candidate in cultural studies and comparative literature at the University of Minnesota. She has edited *Feminismo y teoría del discurso* (1990) and *Teoría feminista y teoría fílmica* (forthcoming).